PRAISE FOR *THI*

Jennifer Swantkowski's book, 7 ... ...
come perspective on the injuries c ... ...azepines and
other psychiatric medications. She ...ares the practical guidance
to get you through the process of tapering these medications
and supports that process with her psychological insights as a
therapist. *The Waiting Room* offers hope and guidance for those
on the courageous journey of medication withdrawal. These
cornerstones will provide you with the encouragement you need
to become medication free.

Karol Ward, LCSW
Author of *Worried Sick* and *Find Your Inner Voice*

The Waiting Room is a significant contribution to the discussion
on the dangers of this country's casual prescribing habits. Written
with intimacy, deep intelligence, and the eye of a therapist, *The
Waiting Room* is both cautionary tale and generous guide for
those seeking to get off psychotropic medication.

Melissa Bond
Author of *Blood Orange Night*

With a warm and engaging voice, Jennifer Swantkowski shares
her lived experience with prescribed medication injury and
withdrawal. Using her training as a therapist, she shares insights
on coping mentally with the array of debilitating symptoms that
can occur in these conditions. The overall message is one of hope

and healing. This book is a must read for anyone who has been "benched" from medication injury and other forms of chronic illness.

Christy Huff, M.D.
Director, Benzodiazepine Information Coalition

Jennifer Swantkowski has courageously shared her turbulent journey from being a prominent, successful therapist and productive citizen to being suddenly plunged into a living nightmare and trauma caused by medication injury and benzodiazepine withdrawal. This is a beautifully written and sensitive account of how to nurture and guide yourself through an experience of complete hopelessness and despair by seeking knowledge, wisdom, understanding, connection, acceptance, self-compassion, and determination to foster self-healing. It is written from the heart and can be a roadmap for others going through a sudden loss of health or medically induced trauma. *The Waiting Room* is a must-read for those experiencing benzodiazepine withdrawal. In Jennifer's journey, one can find themselves.

Paige Pradko, LPC

When someone is going through benzo withdrawal the one thing they want and need is a professional who understands and has compassion for what they are going through. I would recommend *The Waiting Room* to anyone going through benzo withdrawal as well as their family and support system. I love Jennifer's style of writing; it's as if you are sitting with a therapist who, through her own first-hand knowledge and lived experience, is compassionately walking with you and guiding you through the withdrawal process. This is a must read for all therapists and medical/mental health professionals as it offers a clear understanding of the all too common experience of suffering created by medications and their discontinuation.

Geraldine Burns
Host of podcast *Benzodiazepine*
Awareness With Geraldine Burns

This is a book that shouldn't have to be written. After more than six decades of commercial benzodiazepine availability, it seems reasonable to expect that research communities would have clearly defined boundaries on initiation, limitations on duration of use, and discontinuation glide paths absent most of the actual reported agony. It seems reasonable to expect that medical communities *not* exhibit eyes wide shut by prescribing without informed consent, followed by discrediting and disparaging the agonies reported during medication discontinuation in words and inflections that smack of and stigmatize with accusatory psychosomatic self-culpability. No wonder tens of thousands of benzodiazepine survivors flock to online communities of similarly affected persons to find answers.

In *The Waiting Room*, Jennifer Swantkowski has given us a great gift: a master class on how she has and others might negotiate not only the nonlinear and imperfect journey through and beyond the clawed clutches of benzodiazepines, but also through the enormous difficulties posed by doubting clinicians who invalidate lived experiences. How, indeed, can one address the "smelly intruder" that is this medication and its angry, reactive receptors? Can one ever accommodate to this unwelcome visitor that won't leave and remains unrecognized by medical providers who are supposed to acknowledge and assist in the restoration of health? Is radical acceptance possible whereby this caustic trespasser transforms into companion, advisor, and dare I say, friend?

To those affected by benzodiazepines, the author's narrative will resonate strongly, suggests options for scenarios encountered along the way, and provides hope at the end of the day. To benzodiazepine prescribers, Dr. Swantowski's gift includes replacing an old medical cosmology – one that still fundamentally revolves around medical provider at the center of decision-making – with a new one inclusive of right-sized expertise of authentically and fully-involved patients. And to all, she calls us to proceed deliberately, respectfully at "the speed of wisdom" – prudently slower than reactive symptoms and our culture otherwise seem to demand.

Unfortunately, this book had to be written. Fortunately, it is wonderfully done. Read on, then add your own chapters and your own understandings. It's time.

Steven Wright, MD

In *The Waiting Room*, Jennifer Swantkowski offers an engrossing first-person account of her own journey through an adverse medication reaction and prescription medication withdrawal. She not only shares the physical and mental symptoms of the ordeal, but shines a much-needed light on the psychological and emotional challenges that result from those symptoms and from being gaslit by much of the traditional medical community.

Ultimately, Jennifer's book is a useful and encouraging guide for anyone tapering prescription medications and/or working to heal through adverse-reaction or withdrawal situations. She takes readers through coping strategies that have proven helpful for herself and others, and she wisely takes an active approach to healing. Her approach is one that realizes the enormous value of time in the process but also seeks to pursue spiritual and personal growth. Jennifer preaches truth by encouraging readers to find healing through increased faith, hope, gratitude, purpose, balance, and physical health. Also, her book is jam-packed with healing and wellness resources that should prove invaluable to those looking to find their own way forward: websites, books, videos, and counseling referrals. *The Waiting Room* is a must-read "healing companion" for anyone whose life has been complicated by prescription medications.

Michael Priebe,
Writer and Coach at The Lovely Grind

The Waiting Room

My Recovery Journey from Medication Injury
& Benzodiazepine Withdrawal

By Jennifer Swantkowski, PhD, LCSW

The Waiting Room

Copyright © 2022 by Jennifer Swantkowski, PhD.

ISBN: 979-8-9860523-0-4

First edition.

Author website: www.jenniferswanphd.com

Disclaimer:

The Waiting Room is meant for informational and educational purposes only. It is not intended to be used as specific clinical or medical advice or to be used as a replacement for seeking out your own clinical and medical care/advice.

I am not endorsing or recommending any therapists, coaches, philosophies, ideologies, or modalities of treatment. I offer these only in the telling of my journey and to punctuate what has both aided and/or disrupted my own healing process.

THE WAITING ROOM

CHAPTER ONE

THE PROBLEM

"If the only tool you have is a hammer,
you will start treating all your problems like a nail."

- Abraham Kaplan (modified by Abraham Maslow)

I want to start by being clear that this is *not* a book against "Big Pharma." Nor is it an attack on physicians or the medical establishment. Several of my closest friends are doctors. My uncle is a gastroenterologist, and my mom is a nurse. I had a grandma with diabetes treated successfully with insulin. I grew up without worrying about polio, tetanus, or a host of other illnesses. I have many friends who have navigated and survived various cancers over the years and loved ones with high blood pressure and other ailments. I absolutely see the value in medication and am enormously grateful for the major medical advances over the years.

However, my personal experience having a medication-induced injury has certainly shaped me into being incredibly mindful about rushing to traditional medications too quickly to rid myself of aches, pains, and ailments. It has also opened my mind to a wide array of alternative approaches to health care, intervention, and maintenance. I grew up in the era where you listened and blindly followed the dictum of doctors, teachers, and parents. If Walter Cronkite said it on the nightly news, then it must be true. If Mom or Dad said, "Because I said so," that was the end of it. And if my doctor said, "Take this pill," I complied. While a part of me still longs for the *here's all you need to know* simplicity of the Cronkite era, I am forever changed regarding putting my health and life in the hands of anyone without fully investigating other possible options and potential outcomes. That includes making sure I have all the data for fully informed consent and looking at options and discourse that may exist beyond the more mainstream, conventional medical model of care.

Unfortunately, for virtually all medications, there are side effects. We've all seen the ads on TV with the litany of possible side effects, potential reactions, etc. Listen to these, please. Ask questions. *Gas with oily discharge* was always a potential side effect I would hear about on TV as a young adult. I would laugh and think, *Oh no!* If I remember correctly, I think it was a weight loss medication. I would think, *So you are skinny but leak oil out of your butt. No thanks!* But while gas with oily discharge may be embarrassing, things like *potential and possibly permanent effects to your central nervous system* (the one that got me) can leave you a shell of who you once were. So, yes, most medications have side effects, and usually, the pros outweigh the cons. However, most meds also have the unlucky people who have a dramatic and adverse reaction to the medication, who I will unscientifically refer to as the *three-to-five percenters.*

It is important to note that 3-5% is purely a percentage I pulled out of my you know where. I don't know that we have true, accurate rates of adverse effects from antibiotics and other medications because so many are either not reported or the adverse effects are diagnosed as separate issues and treated with more medications. However, regarding benzodiazepine (most common are Xanax, Klonopin, Ativan, Valium, and Librium) withdrawal, the Benzo Information Coalition cites various statements and studies indicating 40-80% of people will experience withdrawal symptoms, with 40% experiencing moderate to severe symptoms. A certain percentage of these individuals will go on to experience protracted withdrawal in which the withdrawal symptoms can last from months to years post cessation of the medication. In 2020, the U.S. Center for Health Statistics reported that 66 million doctor appointments each year result in the prescription of a benzodiazepine. Keep in mind that these statistics were calculated by looking at years 2014 through 2016. PRE-COVID! I can only imagine what this will look like as more recent statistics are available. If we go with a very conservative number and say that only 5% of individuals taking benzodiazepines experience severe withdrawal and/or protracted withdrawal symptoms, then using the above-mentioned stat, that would equate to 3.5 million Americans each year. Even if we went with a ridiculously low number of 1%, we are still talking about over half a million Americans that could be inflicted with a life-altering withdrawal experience. The late Dr. Heather Ashton, Professor Emeritus at The University of New Castle upon Tyne and author of the *Ashton Manual*, and others have collected well over 200 possible symptoms associated with withdrawal and protracted withdrawal that range from tinnitus and insomnia to homicidal and suicidal ideation/completion.

Regardless, those of us with adverse medication effects or complicated discontinuation experiences tend to be seen as the *outliers*. While 3-5% seems low, if you fall in that tiny, marginal portion of the population, being in that cohort becomes 100% a problem. Your problem. Still, 5% (maybe less, maybe more) are good odds, especially when treating cancer, heart disease, and lung or kidney failure. Most would take those odds; I still would.

The insult to injury wasn't that I realized that I landed in that unlucky minority. My struggles were the realization that the medication I had been prescribed, a fluoroquinolone antibiotic, was not appropriate given my ailment of a sore throat and a cough. The side effects and potential adverse reactions were never discussed with me to allow for full informed consent. When I did exhibit a terrible reaction, I was dismissed and made to feel like an overly anxious, histrionic hypochondriac. My current struggle has been further complicated as I work to safely navigate a complicated benzodiazepine withdrawal, which is still widely misunderstood and often discarded in the medical community. Thus, re-opening the wound of feeling unseen, being cast into medical no-man's land yet again, and working hard to maintain my sense of reality and dignity while navigating this controversial terrain. This is what I refer to as the *secondary trauma* of my experience.

There is what happened to me, and then there is how what happened to me was managed and received by others. Being dismissed and made to feel crazy—my debilitating issues were written off by more than seven different specialists—was by far the worst part of my nightmare. Then to find myself years later on the same battlefield/different drug has been exhausting and, at times, demoralizing.

I almost titled this book *When Good Meds Turn Bad.* This is an important point to clarify because the meds I will be discussing that resulted in my central nervous system injury are not in and of themselves bad medicines. In fact, I am sure they have helped many more than they have hurt. That said, the manner in which they are prescribed, without full informed consent, and/or for much longer periods of time than the FDA deems safe and discontinued is problematic. I believe more than tens of thousands of people each year are losing months and years of their lives while suffering the consequences. I hope that as we continue to tell our stories, the ever-growing piles of anecdotal evidence will finally capture the medical community's attention and lead to a much-needed change in the way the meds are prescribed and discontinued.

In many ways, writing this has been a cathartic experience for me—painful and emotional at many turns along the way. I hope that sharing this traumatic health narrative and the skills and tools I obtained and continue to learn along the way will touch another who may be reading these words thinking, *There is no hope.* There is; please keep reading.

My story will be told in two parts, chronicling two distinct episodes. While there was certainly not a full recovery between the two episodes, enough was going well that I felt I had healed. This journey began for me in September 2016, and the first episode lasted until around August 2017. The second episode occurred in late December of 2019, and even as I write, I am still managing many symptoms and issues. Before I jump in, let me start by sharing some background about me and my life before September of 2016, focusing on more salient points regarding my mental and physical health.

Prior to September 2016, I was a healthy, high-functioning woman who worked intensely, loved fully, and moved through life relatively well. My closest friends would probably have described me as an *over-functioner,* and I don't think they were wrong. Being a caregiver was in my blood.

I had worked hard as a clinician for over 20 years and loved what I did. Choosing to get a Master's in Social Work at the age of 25 and then eventually moving on to complete a PhD, I enjoyed all of the various experiences my field offered. This included working in children and adult hospice; developing trauma groups; teaching at Boston College and the University of Houston; working as a family therapist at the Austen Riggs Center; teaching and working as an individual and family therapist at The Menninger Clinic, as well as my own private practice.

When 2016 hit, I was solely focused on my private practice and thought, *This is the year I am going to finally write that book*—a dream I have held since I was a teenager. Don't look for that book; you won't find it. I'd like to blame the inability to finish it on what happened with my health, but what holds more truth is that the book's lack of existence has more to do with me—just me and my avoidance, procrastination, and resistance. The things I would occupy myself with to NOT write were fascinating. Suddenly I needed to reorganize my office, take up a hobby, or bury myself in any task that wasn't writing.

From a personal perspective, I had been a caregiver in my family of origin and channeled much of my energy into the folks that I love as they navigated unique and traumatic losses and subsequent grieving processes. I had a large, loyal group of friends and came from a very large family. My favorite words then (and now) were/are: *Aunt Jen.*

I wasn't taking any medications other than a thyroid med that I had been on since the age of twenty. I am not going to say there weren't times my work and personal commitments didn't lead to mental fatigue, some stress-induced aches, pains, and issues throughout the years. They did. But I would bounce back quickly and resume my high-functioning life. As stressful or tiring as things might be at times, I was always incredibly grateful for my career, my family, and my friends. I felt blessed. Looking back, did I live from an attitude of gratitude all the time? No, not really. I, like many, ran through life occasionally giving the thumbs up to God or thinking, *I have so much to be grateful for*, but life would take over, and I would forget to slow down and pay attention to the daily gifts.

Then life stepped in on that fateful September day, dropped me to my knees, and forced me to slow down. Hell, forget slow down. It threw me down, sucker-punched me, and stood over me with a menacing glare while daring me to just try to get up. As a dear person in my life said to me, knowing my love of all-things sports (and all things JJ Watt), "You've been benched, Jen."

CHAPTER TWO
EPISODE ONE – SEPTEMBER 2016

"What fresh hell can this be?"

- Dorothy Parker

It was a hot, sticky Friday in Houston. I had not felt well for a few days—run-down, scratchy throat, and a slight headache. I took a few Ibuprofen and powered through, ready to see the seven clients I had scheduled for the day. However, halfway through, I realized I had run out of juice.

I called and canceled my last few sessions of the day. My throat was hurting, my head pounding, and I felt feverish. Being early afternoon on a Friday, it was impossible to see my internist immediately, so I decided just to go home and take the weekend to relax and heal.

As I drove home, I felt worse with each minute that passed. I wasn't sure if it was the flu. Maybe strep throat? Could just be a bad sinus infection. I decided to stop by an urgent care center near my house. I was seen almost immediately, and after a few minutes with the doctor, he felt I might have the beginning of bronchitis. I told him I would see my internist as soon as possible the following week.

However, he felt it would be good to get on top of it and wrote me two prescriptions—one for an antibiotic, the generic version of the antibiotic Levaquin called Levofloxacin, and an oral steroid. Since I had previously not done well on steroids, I chose not to fill that script. This proved serendipitous, and I thanked God when I learned later that taking a steroid with this particular type of antibiotic can cause big issues for certain people. I have since learned that taking a benzodiazepine while on this class of antibiotics can strip the GABA-A receptor leading to acute benzo withdrawal. I also learned, unfortunately much too late, that combining NSAIDS (Motrin, Advil, etc.) with this particular antibiotic was also highly problematic for many. I was never asked at the urgent care center if I was on any of these medications. While I wasn't on a benzo, I had most certainly been taking loads of NSAIDs earlier in the day and throughout the short time taking the antibiotic. I will never know if that led to the adverse reactions coming my way.

I filled the antibiotic prescription, went home, and took the first pill. It was 6:00 p.m. I fell asleep early, and woke up in middle of the night dizzy and sweating and felt like I was getting worse. I was thankful for the antibiotic as I assumed my new symptoms of dizziness, blurred vision, and vacillating from burning to freezing resulted from my illness. I woke up the next morning on the cold tile floor of the bathroom having no memory of how I had gotten there. I ate breakfast and took my second dose.

I remember starting to feel like I was going to have a panic attack, which I attributed to being so sick and worried about my busy week ahead. I felt too ill to begin calling my Monday patients to cancel and prayed that I would be feeling better and wouldn't have to do so by Sunday.

I took my third and what turned out to be my final dose that evening. That Saturday night, I mostly tossed and turned as I came in and out of what I describe as *toxic sleep*. The next morning, I woke up, and my ears began to scream. Sounds dramatic because it was. My ears began to literally scream a high-pitched squeal that would not stop. I began to pace my home, sweating and freezing, feeling like my eyesight had suddenly and dramatically changed, as everything was blurry.

I couldn't sit still, and I felt as if someone had plugged me into a socket. As I paced my home, I began to feel a sense of fear that I had never experienced before. I looked in the mirror and wondered if I was real. There were moments I did not recognize myself or my home. I looked through the window at the backyard and saw the pool. Suddenly the thought that I would drown myself in the pool was upon me. I was not suicidal and never had been. I did not feel depressed. In fact, I did not feel *real* enough to even have a mood state. It was an intrusive thought that I would simply drown myself in the swimming pool. I immediately double-locked the door. Some small part of me was still intact—the objective, healthy "me" trying to protect myself from going into the backyard.

I called a dear friend who is a psychiatrist and oversees an inpatient hospital unit and said, "I think you need to hospitalize me—something is very wrong." My friend stayed on the phone with me for nearly two hours, and I slightly began to come back into myself. We agreed that since the only thing that had changed was taking a new medication, I should stop the antibiotic until I could see my internist on Monday. This gem of a human and a few other friends were my lifelines along the way.

I went to splash cold water on my face and was met with the intrusive thought, *You could just drown yourself in the bathtub or even this sink.* Suddenly, and for the next two weeks, any sight of water led me to a series of strange, intrusive thoughts. Stranger, though, is that I have zero fear of the water. I was a swimmer, and I feel my best in the water. Never in my 46 years had I ever experienced an intrusive thought or ever been suicidal. Even though my identity as a psychotherapist was the furthest thing from my mind in these moments, I was learning something about fear, annihilation anxiety, and a distrust of one's mind that would have a profound impact on the way I sat with and understood my clients in the future.

I was aware there was still some sliver of me observing this rapid mental and physical deterioration of myself. Some part of me that was able to say, *This isn't you. Something has happened to you. You just need to stay safe.* That evening I laid myself down to sleep, and my legs and arms burned as though someone was holding one of those three-foot-long, gray, Fourth of July sparklers against them. I began to have shooting pains in my feet and calves, my screaming ears had dulled to a constant whooshing sound, and I was unable to see well enough to watch TV or read.

I tried to play some of my favorite music. I found Chris Botti on my phone only to realize I suddenly had developed Spidey ears (also known as hyperacusis) and could not tolerate music even at its lowest volume. Then the pacing resumed, back and forth between the kitchen and the bedroom. I had no idea how to quell the intense internal tremor or calm my mind. And that night, having never experienced insomnia before, became the longest night's journey into day I could ever imagine.

On Monday morning, having been out of bed pacing since 4:00 a.m. in the morning, I was so grateful for the break of dawn. Being unable to rest while the world slept intensified my fear and distress. I was unable to look in the mirror as I only saw a distortion, and what was reflected back to me was unrecognizable. I would pinch myself to keep myself in the moment and not drift into an altered state of consciousness.

I could not wait to hear back from my internist and somehow got in my car and drove the 11 miles to her office. I sat in the parking lot from 7:00 a.m. until they opened at 8:00 a.m. I walked in feeling like I possibly needed to and feared that I would be sent immediately to the emergency room, or worse, a locked psych ward.

It was all surreal. I do not remember how I got past the front desk into a room waiting to see my doctor. The internist I had seen for five years had recently retired, and I had only met her replacement on one brief occasion for a yearly physical. As I waited and paced the office, I thought, *Pull it together, Jen.* She entered the room, and I tried my best to sound somewhat coherent as I rattled off my list of symptoms. Although I remember her to be kind, I am quite certain she distrusted me, believing instead that I was a closet alcoholic, drug seeker, or just very mentally disturbed. I described the tinnitus, the shooting pains, the blurry vision, the elephant on my chest, the pressure in my head, feelings of not being real, an inability to concentrate, and insomnia as she typed them all into the computer. Eventually, she turned and looked at me. I realized I was pacing and forced myself to sit down. We were both quiet for what seemed an eternity.

She took my pulse and said she was happy I had discontinued the antibiotic. She asked several questions: had I been drinking on it, doing drugs, taking other antibiotics? All were a big *no*. She said the medication might still be in my system, but felt sure that what I was experiencing wasn't related to the antibiotic. Without looking at me, she said, "Have you ever been diagnosed with Generalized Anxiety Disorder? That would explain most of this."

I began to cry.

Of course, looking back, that probably only strengthened the narrative I feared she was creating in her mind: a middle-aged hysteric.

I fought my way back to a moment of sanity and said, "Please, I need you to hear me. I have no psychiatric history. Yes, I have had my share of stressors and probably could have managed these stressors better in my life. I am on no medications, nor have I ever taken any other than my thyroid med for hypothyroidism that I have had since I was twenty. But I just had blood work a month ago, and that has been stable for many years. I work a lot. I have a vibrant private practice. I love what I do. I am very active. Last week I had a sore throat and took this prescribed medication. Today, I no longer recognize myself."

Perhaps this moment of clarity slowed her down a bit. She actually looked at me for a long time and said, "It is clear you are in a lot of distress. Let's get you in to see some specialists and get some blood work right away."

Over the next four days, as I waited to see the neurologist, my blood work came back. I'll never forget the nurse calling me and saying, "Good news, your blood work is just fine—except, funny thing, you are now hyperthyroid, so you are going to have to get into your endocrinologist and get that taken care of."

I asked to speak to the doctor. Later that day, when the doctor called back, I asked, "Don't you think it's strange that a month ago my thyroid labs were stable, had been for many years, and now suddenly, and for the first time in my life, I am hyperthyroid?"

She said, "Jennifer, most of your symptoms could be explained by hyperthyroidism. We may have found the answer."

I hung up and cried again. I would have LOVED for it to have been that simple. *But we know our bodies.* No matter how crazy you are made to feel, do not ever forget that you are the one wearing that bag of skin, and you know it better than anyone.

I saw seven specialists over the next 24 days: cardiologists, neurologists, endocrinologists, gastroenterologists, ENTs, an OB-GYN, and my internist. I won't bore you with all the details, but what I heard over and over again was some version of this: "Jennifer, I don't really know what is happening, but I know it can't be the antibiotic. It is long out of your system."

I recall saying many times, "I'm aware it's out of my system, but is it possible that while it was in my system, it caused some sort of damage?"

A few told me that they heard about spontaneous tendon ruptures caused by this med, but nothing like I was describing. Each and every one of them recommended I see a psychiatrist and look at depression and anxiety disorders. *So, this med could cause your Achilles heel to spontaneously rupture, but it was too much of a leap to think that it could potentially cause other damage?*

In the three months that followed that fateful September day, I would see seven specialists and have a total of over 25 doctor's appointments.

One of my *favorite* appointments came two months later when the endocrinologist, who had pulled me off all my thyroid meds (the first time in 26 years), said, "Well, the good news is you no longer have a thyroid situation. Your bloodwork has been normal for six weeks. No more meds for you, at least for now. We will check again in six months." Keep in mind as he said this, I was still not sleeping, had lost 17 pounds, had returned to work but at a reduced capacity, and would return home only to pace and try to find ways to manage the screaming in my ears, the tremor in my chest, and the pain in my legs.

I looked at him and said, "Okay, but wait, don't you at least find this interesting? I've had hypothyroid since I was 20 years old, and I've been on medications for the last 26 years. I took an antibiotic, I feel like a bomb went off inside me, and suddenly I am cured?"

As he patted my shoulder and opened the door to walk out, he said, "I didn't say cured. We will see in six months, but for now, go and celebrate."

That was the moment.

The moment where I felt something in me crack. I had gone through life and had never really felt a full-frontal impact of being disavowed, disbelieved, devalued, invisible, or written off as *crazy* or *unstable.* Unfortunately, this blessing meant that I had no skill set to help me manage or make sense of how to maneuver a world in which I was now being overtly written off, unseen, unheard, and pathologized. While I didn't know it then, this too would forever change me in my clinical practice and in my life. The sheer rage, disorientation, and hopelessness caused by that sort of gaslighting is something I will take to my grave. And the pain opened me up to an awareness that has forever changed how I think about all sorts of marginalized or disempowered individuals and groups. I had always been a social worker in thought, heart, and career choice, but this trauma drilled further in me a need to always search for one's humanity, to really listen, and to trust that maybe not seeing or understanding something did not mean it was not true or didn't exist. This secondary trauma of being written off, while nearly breaking me emotionally, is what ultimately led me to discover and become a lover of the philosophy of Stoicism, deepen my faith, develop mental strategies to increase resilience, and led to the realization that it was up to me to fight for my health and recovery. This is not to say that I didn't have loving, caring friends, colleagues, and family that were pulling for me. However, I was out there in medical no-man's land, and you have to go through that part of the journey alone.

As I slumped out of the endocrinologist's office to *celebrate*, feeling the worst possible pain I could imagine, I began to laugh. I climbed into my car and laughed a crazy, maniacal, carnival laugh. Imagine Tom Hank's character Walter Fielding in *The Money Pit*. He is standing over a hole in the floor after the bathtub that he was filling with a bucket falls through to the living room below, belting out a crazy, carnival laugh while his life and home fall to pieces around him. That was me in my Pathfinder, laughing and crying like a sad, dysregulated party clown.

However, in that laugh, I remembered something—a bit of me. I had been a funny person. I had been a good aunt and a loving daughter, a vested therapist, a kind sibling, and a caring friend. I was going to come out of this. This is when a few things began to turn around for me. Not physically—that would be many, many months later—but psychologically, I felt *me* reach out for me (if that makes sense) and wrap my arms around myself. I remember sitting in my car thinking, *I am going to be okay*.

I recalled one of my lovely clients telling me about the Stockdale Paradox. James Stockdale had been a prisoner of war, and when asked how he survived mentally and physically, he said he didn't hold out false hope like, *I'll be home by Christmas.*

He would say to himself something like this: *I am going to be okay, one day. I don't know when that is, but today is obviously not that day, and today, I have to do what I need to do to survive this hell.* As I sat in my car shaking, scared, and feeling a thousand miles away from who I had been just a few months before, I thought, *You will be okay, but today is not that day. For now, you need to do what needs to be done.* This system of reasonable hope and radical acceptance has become very handy over the years.

Although I knew I hadn't developed a crippling form of anxiety overnight, and most of the emotional and mental symptoms had begun to dissipate, I knew the symptoms that remained were causing a great deal of distress. I needed to find someone willing to try to help me. I had exhausted nearly all other specialties, so I decided to find a good psychiatrist to see if they could help me find any answers. Having worked with and befriended many good psychiatrists in the Houston area over the years in my profession, I chose one I deeply respected but didn't run in my circle of friends.

This doctor had also never known this antibiotic to cause these symptoms, but he believed I had been injured by it. We started to treat the symptoms with nerve medication (gabapentin) and a common benzodiazepine (alprazolam, the generic of Xanax) to slow down what appeared to be symptoms of a wildly sensitized nervous system: neuropathy, tinnitus, fuzzy vision, nausea, difficulty sleeping, and shooting, random nerve pain throughout my body. Again, all of this was well-meaning, but I would learn years later it was not a good fit for me.

I was still nowhere close to my baseline, but I was starting to notice better hours, better days. My clients and my nieces and nephews got all I had to give. I would go home and pace; put in my ear plugs to manage my hyperacusis (Spidey ears); stare in terror at my bedroom that had become a house of horrors; still only get three to four hours of sleep a night before being jolted awake by a storm of adrenaline and cortisol; and experience racing thoughts and fear that I would never again be okay.

As time went on, I made a game out of the random piercing pains in my feet and legs—like a bad game of whack-a-mole—where would the next one pop up? After having my vision checked twice, I began to accept the feeling of wearing fogged-up goggles (the one symptom that has never left) as just being part of my new life.

Then in early January 2017, four months after the antibiotic injury, two things happened that were crucial to my healing. First, I went to see a new ENT regarding the overwhelming tinnitus and hyperacusis. He listened to me and said, "Oh my God, I think I know what happened. My wife went through this. I think you had a neurotoxic reaction to the antibiotic."

He explained that although my reaction was rare, there was an existing Black Box warning on all of the fluoroquinolone antibiotics since 2008, warning against spontaneous tendon ruptures. He explained it had been amended again in 2013, advising that this class of medication could cause potentially irreversible neuropathy (nerve damage). In 2015, a Federal Advisory Council meeting deemed the risks outweighed the benefits of using fluoroquinolones (Levaquin, Cipro, etc.) for sinusitis, urinary tract infections, and bronchitis (I was placed on it for possible bronchitis). Then, it was amended again in 2016 (five months before I was injured), adding the warning for potentially serious, disabling, and permanent side effects that could involve: the tendons, muscles, joints, nerves, and central nervous system. I remember feeling both vindicated and sick to my stomach simultaneously. I told him that I had been to seven specialists and over two dozen doctor's visits in the last few months and had been told by each that the antibiotic could not be responsible for the myriad of symptoms.

I remember he looked down and said, "I honestly don't know. It's hard to keep up with all of the changes of every medication, but your symptoms are clearly that of an injury to the nervous system, so why they didn't slow down and dig deeper… I just don't know."

The following words were a game-changer for me, "Jennifer, I am so sorry this happened to you. You should never have been given this medication. It's a very heavy antibiotic, a hard hitter, not meant for a sore throat. Maybe if you'd tried several other antibiotics with no relief or had severe pneumonia and were in the hospital, but you probably had a bad cold. This medication should be used as a last resort. At the very least, you should have been informed of the risks." I could literally feel the effects of being seen, heard, and understood. I could feel my resolve strengthen in his words and gaze.

Later that same week, I decided I would try to do something

normal other than going to work and home again. I went and got my hair cut and colored. Having normally been in every four to six weeks, my regular hairdresser said, "Girl, where have you been?"

I was used to not sharing the truth about how I was currently doing, as I feared being disbelieved or seen as a hypochondriac. But for some reason, I decided to be open and honest. I said, "Well, I've actually been really sick. It's kind of a long story, but basically, I took this antibiotic—a generic form of Levaquin. And it kind of blew up my life!" I am sure my voice broke.

I think, sensing my distress, Stephanie touched my shoulder and said, "Wait, don't say anything else—let me tell you something first." She explained that about a year earlier, she had been going out of town to go surfing and got sick and was started on a generic version of Levaquin.

She described not feeling great on it and having a bad headache. On the fourth day of her seven-day prescription, she took Ibuprofen to help with her headache. She said, "Jen, I jolted out of bed a couple of hours later. My heart was racing; I was having a panic attack." She went on to describe a litany of my own symptoms, including issues with blurry vision, floaters, strange pains, rapid onset panic attacks (with no prior history), and a sense of feeling detached and dissociative. She, like me, had tried to figure out what could have caused these things to happen.

I sat there with my mouth open as she described a parallel process to the hell I had been in for months. I could have jumped up and hugged her. I told her how many doctors and health professionals had told me that my issues were *an underlying anxiety condition* and were not associated with the antibiotic, as they felt it was long out of my system.

Between the ENT doctor and Stephanie's validation, I felt another shift in my psychological attitude towards myself and my struggle. I knew I wasn't crazy, but it felt so incredibly important to have found someone who could mirror and validate that for me. I had found a trauma twin in Stephanie, and no longer feeling alone made an enormous difference.

Soon, I found a few online support groups and discovered that my condition was referred to as being *floxed*, as in an injury caused by the group of fluoroquinolone antibiotics. I was horrified to find literally thousands of people suffering far more debilitating reactions than myself. I eventually had to literally step away and stop reading the terrifying stories of people, young and old, talking about being bedbound, needing multiple surgeries to correct torn tendons, and many, like me, who were suffering from neurological issues for years with no remission.

I knew I couldn't allow myself to get swallowed up in the horror of it all, and I had to pray I would be one of the lucky ones and focus on positive thoughts and actions.

With my alprazolam and my gabapentin on board, I just treated my symptoms and worked hard to move forward in my life as best I could. At the time, my doctor and I didn't know that we were, quite possibly, creating another issue for me down the road with this mix of medications. This was somewhat unchartered territory, and we were both just trying to take it one day at a time. His belief that there had been an adverse reaction and his desire to stay with me through it was invaluable. We didn't know if my nervous system was injured or damaged, so we just did the best we could, and I prayed that it would eventually resolve.

In time, it did. I was significantly better five to six months later, and I really turned a corner around month eight or nine. I began to take the medications less and less, knowing nothing about withdrawal or how to come off these meds. Did I mention I had been in the field of psychology/psychiatry for 24 years at this time? Yep, and I didn't know that most people need to taper off these meds very slowly to avoid a rough withdrawal. It took a lot of work on self-compassion to forgive myself for not knowing. By the first anniversary date, I was rarely taking them, only as needed, and I fought taking them at all. By month 15, I was off them altogether.

Withdrawal from benzos is not an easy, smooth process for many, and many do not do well with the standard procedure of cutting it down by 25% every few weeks. But amazingly, I did. I simply walked off them. This stroke of luck would prove to be disastrous, as it is for many, as I didn't think twice about taking a benzodiazepine again when it was prescribed to me during my second episode a few years later.

While significantly better, I had not returned to my baseline. I was very functional, worked full time, and was able to be an aunt, sister, and friend while loving, playing, and being fully in my life. However, my eyes were always blurry; I still dealt with tinnitus several times a month; and I could just tell that my *innards* seemed to be just a bit more fragile. I felt like I was propped up with toothpicks and bubblegum rather than the titanium posts that had once held me up.

So, what did I do? I wanted to distance myself far, far away from that woman who had become so ill. To move past how close I had come to losing my mind and nearly losing myself. I did not want to look back. I did not want to research too much. A part of me wanted to return to the *floxed* sites to let my suffering comrades know there was light at the end of the tunnel. But I couldn't. When I would log on and see the train wreck the antibiotic had left in the lives of so many, I would feel a need to run far away and pretend that I had not just dodged a very lethal bullet.

I had to log off. I wanted only to look forward. I had been one of the lucky ones. And with an element of survivor's guilt, I trudged on.

The next two-and-a-half years had their own share of stressors and joys. My life has always gone that way — love big, hurt big. Big joys, big losses. With an immediate family of 20 members and growing larger by the year, there was always so much to keep us entertained or crisis managed.

Health-wise, I was doing fine. I worked hard to stay well and was terrified of ever taking an antibiotic again. I knew I would never return to a fluoroquinolone but had also developed a strong fear of most medications.

I was back to traveling to New York City several times a year to quench my thirst for all-things musical theater. I was going out with friends, hosting parties, had moved into a beautiful new apartment in my favorite part of Houston, and my private practice was thriving. I was enjoying weekend slumber parties with my various nieces and nephews, attending their sporting events, and going on family vacations. I got to watch one of the pieces of my heart as she gave her high school salutatorian speech and headed off to Notre Dame. I was happy.

Unfortunately, as fate would have it, the lights in my life were flickering again. My battles with medications were not over.

CHAPTER THREE

EPISODE TWO – DECEMBER 2019

"If you're going through hell, keep going."

- Winston Churchill

In December 2019, three years and three months after the initial event, I had to have minor surgery to remove polyps from my uterus. The surgery took 45 minutes. I woke up and felt GREAT! I went home still feeling wonderful, and I actually told the family members helping me settle in, "I feel like I want to go for a run!" I don't run. Ever. Bad sign.

I tried to calm down, but I soon realized my eyes were more foggy than normal. Within an hour, my ears began to scream, and an internal tremor took over my body. I could see my loved one on the other side of the couch, but I suddenly wasn't sure if they were real—if I was real.

Oh no, I thought. And quickly dismissed the idea that it could be happening again.

Had they given me a fluoroquinolone in my anesthesia cocktail even though it was written all over my chart that I was "allergic?"

After a few days, I reached back out to the wonderful psychiatrist who had helped me years before, and we agreed to return to the old standbys of gabapentin and alprazolam as needed. However, he had left his clinical work to focus on research, and we agreed I needed to look for a new primary doctor to help me through these complications just in case this turned out to be another long-term issue.

I began the meds, but unfortunately, they didn't work this time. The gabapentin almost immediately made me feel awful, but I was advised to take more as my body was clearly not benefitting from the relatively small dosage. *More meds will help,* I thought, agreeing with the advice I was given by many. As the weeks went on, I felt spacey, dizzy, nauseous, disconnected, and just an overall sense of *being off.* By this time, I was without a primary physician to spearhead treatment, and although I had some lovely, well-meaning, and brilliant doctor friends trying to help me as best they could, we all know you can't treat your loved ones or friends. I was so disgusted and upset that this was happening again. I hid my symptoms and kind of went underground, keeping to myself, not sharing how bad things were, ashamed of what was happening, and worried no one could help me. I was increasing the gabapentin and trying to avoid taking the alprazolam (Xanax), as I knew it was a controlled substance, and I feared dependence, even though I had escaped it the first time. I was taking 600mg to 1200mg of gabapentin daily and maybe 0.25mg to 0.5mg of alprazolam if I couldn't sleep. But I could feel my body slipping away from me. My sleep became more erratic. I began to lose weight and struggled to feel well enough to eat. I had stabbing pains in my feet and legs, heart palpitations, and began to develop a pervasive sense of what felt like low-level fear and dread accompanying me constantly.

I changed my diet and went *no sugar*. Did I mention I am an all-or-nothing sort? Yep. So, I went from a sugar fiend to no sugar in a week. I had heard of a Herxheimer reaction, our bodies' natural reaction to detoxification when we give up sugar or caffeine or undergo a formal liver or kidney detox protocol, etc. My body, already weakened from the surgery and the resurgence of my central nervous system issues, was compromised, and the radical diet change sent me over the edge.

I sat in my sessions with clients with a heating pad on my hands to manage the intense temperature dysregulations in my body. I would get through my day and go home, only to land on the couch and stare off into space for a couple of hours. After a couple of months, I stopped the gabapentin cold turkey. I had no idea this was a medication that needed a slow-taper to come off effectively. (Some are able to walk off as I had back in 2016.) I could feel the walls closing in. As I felt less and less in control, I was advised to increase my intake of alprazolam. It worked until it didn't.

Within a few weeks, I thought I was losing my mind. By this time, I had increased my dose to 0.5mg twice per day, but I was feeling worse and worse. I wanted this drug out of my system and tried to come off by dropping the dose by around 25-30% in a ten-day period. I felt like I was losing my grip on reality. The world suddenly seemed large and distorted, and I struggled at times to recognize myself in the mirror. After ten days of pure hell, and per the advice I was given, I up-dosed to a much larger dose of 1.5mg per day.

I finally got in to see my new psychiatrist, but I was a shell of myself by then. I was shaky, terrified, and kept thinking, *I know I am in some sort of withdrawal or having a negative reaction. I need to get off this stuff.*

This new doctor was very kind, but again, did not seem to understand what was happening to me fully. He said I appeared incredibly anxious, and it was clear I was struggling mightily. His strong recommendation was to increase the dose rather than try to come off it. The exact statement was, "So what if you end up needing 6mg of this stuff to make you feel better? If that is what you need, that is what you need. Your anxiety about needing to get off is making things worse." Six milligrams? If you don't know, a 6mg dose is a BOAT LOAD of Xanax.

I left and felt that old familiar sense of being alone and possibly seen as an anxious wreck of a human being. I do respect the fact that in my first session, he told me straight away that he wasn't sure he would be able to help me. When doctors tell you that, listen to them. He wasn't being a jerk; he was being sincere. He never heard of a neuro-toxic reaction to fluoroquinolones, and at that point, neither of us understood if my experiences were a continuation of that original injury or something new altogether. But remember, we are the experts on our bodies, we have to listen to ourselves, and I felt strongly this was not JUST a continuation of being *floxed*. I worried I had now entered benzo-hell, and no amount of upping the dose would save me from what I needed to do.

But I stayed. I was desperate. I knew I would hold my ground and not increase my dosage, and he was supportive of my decision. It wasn't the best fit, but he was kind to me, and I felt broken beyond repair. I told myself, *At least he cares.*

However, again, *something* kicked in for me. I was already in therapy (something I have always believed all therapists need to be doing), and it was in my own therapy, facing my own mental and physical demise, that I realized I had to advocate for myself again to find my way out of this mess. My gut told me that it didn't matter if this was a prolonged reaction from being *floxed* years before or not. What I was facing now was a bad reaction to the benzodiazepine and quite possibly an injury from going cold turkey off the gabapentin. It didn't matter if I was the only one on the planet going through this. It was clearly here, and I wasn't sure how long it planned to stay.

I made a plan to close down my private practice. This was, *by far*, the hardest thing I ever had to do. I had worked so hard to create a very successful practice with clients that I deeply cared about. It was a great joy in my life, and I felt blessed every day as I walked into my office. I would think, *I can't believe I get to do what I love.* So, to realize that shutting down was ethically the right decision was devastating. However, I was becoming increasingly more ill and knew if I didn't do it, it would shut itself down.

Within 24 hours of contacting each of my clients, I wasn't able to read. It was like my brain held on just long enough to get me through leaving my beloved clients with a bit of grace and dignity. Then the bottom dropped.

I couldn't read. I couldn't think. I would stand in the kitchen for an hour staring at a sweet potato, and I could not figure out how to heat it up. I stopped eating and lost 26 pounds in 21 days. My mind would race so fast that I felt I was having a manic episode, and I began to have strange distortions of time and space. I often didn't know what month it was, was afraid of my patio, and wondered if perhaps I was a fraud and if I even attended a PhD program. I wondered if maybe I created my entire life story, that none of it was true, and that I would be found out and sent to prison. Strangely, alongside all of these bizarre thoughts, perceptions, and feelings, there was still an intact aspect of myself that was completely aware this was not me. Yet, I could not understand why the thoughts continued to race and loop, why the perceptions continued to distort and haunt me. I wondered if I had done something bad to deserve what was happening to me. I called my family and told them I needed help. I had a lovely apartment in my favorite part of town, an office I was no longer using, and I couldn't think to pay a bill or make a bowl of rice. I was terrified to be alone. The shower became a threatening sight. My own mind felt as if it was turning against me.

I will say that there was a period of about a week (it's all a bit fuzzy) where I truly didn't believe that I would live. All of those strange thoughts continued to crop up and torment me. My brain was betraying me. My own sight of myself was unfamiliar. The people and things I loved the most in the world felt like strangers. My world, and my existence, became utterly terrifying.

So, at the age of 49, I had to accept that I needed around-the-clock care, and I moved back in with my mom and dad. I will never be able to thank them enough for the love they showed me. When I looked at them in pure primal fear, as I sat on the couch trying to listen to a calm podcast, they would mirror back the strong woman they knew instead of the terrified, weak, and sick daughter in front of them.

With the help of my therapist, I came to the conclusion I needed to change doctors. I was afraid. I didn't want to be *that person* that doctor hops. But I wasn't getting better and realized, in part, I didn't feel like my doctor was really interested in digging deeper to find out exactly why I had fallen so far. This was another turning point. I started with a new internist, Dr. B., who believed me and was extremely interested in all that had occurred since 2016. She sat with me for 90 minutes during our first meeting and took copious notes. I also changed psychiatrists. I want to share word-for-word what my new psychiatrist said to me on the day I reached out, as it was another turning point for me. I called Dr. C., having known her professionally as we shared a few clients together. I knew her to be straightforward, clear, and willing to think out-of-the-box. I wasn't sure if she would be comfortable taking me on as a client, but I thank God she did.

After hearing all that had happened, she said, "Jen, you have been through so much. First of all, it seems your nervous system was blown out by the fluoroquinolone, and now it is clear you are struggling with benzo withdrawal. Your system has taken two big hits. Benzodiazepines were never meant for long-term use, and you were lucky the first time to just walk off them. This time, not so much. We need to slow down. We are going to sit right here for a while and build your body back up. We need to focus on nutrition, think about supplementation, and get your body and mind strong enough to tolerate what will, most likely, need to be a very slow and steady taper-off."

This is where the story turns. This is where I find my voice, my strength, and my conviction to heal. This is the moment at which I realized that my study and love of stoicism, my faith, and working on my coping skills would need to be moved from the *important* status in my life to *non-negotiable*. This was the day I got off the proverbial bench and started the slow, steady baby steps into health and healing.

In just a short amount of time, with the newfound confidence of having a supportive mini team of Dr. C., Dr. B., and Sandra (my psychiatrist, my internist, and my therapist, respectively), I began to take an inventory of my symptoms and made my first real attempt at trying to just accept them, despite not knowing if they were temporary or long-term.

There are well over 200 anecdotally noted and documented symptoms reported by people who experienced a complicated benzodiazepine withdrawal. My main symptoms include(d): insomnia; an internal agitation that felt like I was plugged into a nuclear power plant; burning skin; blurry vision; racing thoughts; dark and intrusive thoughts; a constant sense of fear, dread, doom, and gloom; morning terrors; depersonalization and derealization; lack of ability to experience connections to things or people that I love (anhedonia); sensory overstimulation (unable to watch TV, listen to music, or talk on the phone for long periods of time); mental fatigue; a chronic sense of dysphoria; and neuropathy in my legs and feet.

Despite the onslaught of symptoms, I began to stabilize a bit over the next month or so. With the stability came the dawning realization that I had stepped away from something that I loved dearly—being a therapist. Although it had only been a short time, grief set in, and I began second-guessing my decision. The nature of my struggle was that I could have a good day followed by a terrible day or a bad hour followed by a good hour. That said, I knew returning full time, while being erratic and unpredictable, was not something I could do ethically. Interestingly, what happened next was that, suddenly, COVID-19 hit, and all things became virtual in a matter of months.

Several months later, a couple of my clients reached out as they decided not to begin a therapeutic relationship with anyone else once I had left on medical leave. I explained I was in a highly unpredictable health situation and could agree to work with them as needed, so long as they fully understood I could not commit to being as available nor as consistent as I had been or would want to be. With that understanding, I returned to work with a small handful of clients. The promise I made myself, and to them, was that if I were feeling at all *off*, I would not go through with a session. Being fully present and focused was of utmost importance. With this very part-time work, I embarked on the full-time job of balancing symptoms that would often flare with no rhyme or reason, despite my commitment to a *very* slow-and-steady taper off the benzodiazepine.

As I write this, I am less than halfway through my turtle-paced benzodiazepine taper. On my good days, I am 60% myself. On my bad days... well, it isn't pretty. It will be a minimum three-plus-year process of coming off the alprazolam and be free from the med that I took for only a few months. That is not the case for everyone. Many can go much faster. Some have no issues at all. And *many* people struggle mightily, no matter how slowly they come off. Some choose to remain on the benzo as the with-drawal can be tortuous, and *regular life* becomes challenging. But with my team at my side, a plan was formed. We committed to a slow taper and to listen to my body and let it guide us.

Currently, like in 2016, most of my symptoms are *invisible* in nature, and this brings with it a set of unique challenges. I want to stress how important it is, especially when dealing with in-visible illnesses, to have *someone* who believes you. Thank God, I have my mini team, my family, and a few friends who were interested in learning about what had happened to me. This has proven to be invaluable. No one could *see* my blurry vision; bouts of dizziness; stabbing pains in my feet. No one could measure how quickly my body would vacillate from hot to cold. It wasn't easy to understand how one hour I would feel present and the next hour be in a cognitive fog that was so deep, it was terrifying. Nothing showed the waves of chemical depression and anxiety nor the near-constant fear that I would never return to the person I had been.

By the way, I no longer pray for that. I don't want to return to who I once was. Each day, I am growing and transitioning into a new and improved version of myself. Despite the hellish symptoms, I am one of the lucky ones. For many, damages from fluoroquinolone antibiotics have caused permanent disability. For more than tens of thousands trying to come off benzodiazepines, either via taper or having been cut off by their doctor, they describe being bed- and house-bound, unable to work, parent, or function. I will take my whack-a-mole symptoms and my turtle-paced taper any day. Even though my ability to engage, work, and function are quite compromised at times, I learned there may not be a ton to make this better. But it can always get worse. For me, my hope is that going slow will stave off an even worse experience that may happen later without the right care.

If you are interested in learning more about benzodiazepine withdrawal and recovery, there are several excellent resources.

Dr. Steven Wright, MD, served as a primary editor for the book *The Benzodiazepine Crisis: The Ramifications of an Overused Drug Class.* He also co-founded *The Alliance for Benzodiazepines Best Practices* and has done countless interviews on this subject on Sirius XM radio and various podcasts.

Another great resource is the podcast *Benzodiazepine Awareness* by Geraldine Burns, a long-term survivor of benzo withdrawal.

Also, consider listening to the powerful podcast *The Benzo*

Free Podcast by D.E. Foster as well as reading his book *Benzo Free: The World of Anti-Anxiety Drugs and the Reality of Withdrawal.*

I recommend following the story of Dr. Christy Huff, a cardiologist who endured a grueling benzo withdrawal following just weeks of use for a medical condition. Dr. Huff is highly active in advocacy and awareness efforts and is the Director of the Benzodiazepine Information Coalition.

The Council for Evidence-Based Psychiatry out of the UK is also a wealth of information as it seeks to explore existing research and identify gaps in the research regarding psychotropic medications, their efficacy, and prescribing habits.

Nicole Lamberson, a Physician's Assistant, who is vocal about her withdrawal journey, works tirelessly in advocacy and awareness with the Benzodiazepine Information Coalition and is a co-founder of *The Withdrawal Project,* which is part of the Inner Compass Initiative, an online platform whose goal is to increase awareness for better informed consent related to psychiatric medication. Nicole has a multitude of interviews she conducts that are available on their site, and she has been instrumental in the marketing and distribution of the movie *Medicating Normal*— a must see for anyone interested, personally struggling, or has a loved one who is grappling with life-altering symptoms after taking or attempting to come off of a psychiatric medication.

Additionally, filmmaker Holly Hardman has released a documentary feature titled *As Prescribed.* This film not only presents lived experiences of those injured by benzodiazepines, but also spotlights the dogged efforts of benzodiazepine survivor and awareness advocate Geraldine Burns as she leads a charged campaign for informed-consent legislation.

Jocelyn Pedersen's book *Seeds of Hope* and Baylissa Frederick's book *Recovery and Renewal* are also valuable resources that offer personal experience, support, and awareness regarding the depths of benzodiazepine injury.

The list goes on, but I have found some useful nuggets of wisdom in the lives and stories of Jennifer Leigh, David Powers, Chris Paige, Michael Priebe, and Phil Eichinger. Jennifer, David, Michael and Chris are all benzo coaches who offer support to individuals and their families facing complications of benzodiazepine withdrawal. There are various free online support groups made available through Facebook and Benzo Buddies is the largest, world-wide free online support for people affected by benzodiazepines and their loved ones.

Jordan Peterson's daughter has a very chilling but important interview with her father about his horrific withdrawal and recovery experience.

These are just a few of the many important contributions being made every day to the education, awareness, and support for the medical community, people injured by benzodiazepines, and their loved ones. I have listed all these, plus other resources, that have inspired and helped me along in this process at the end of the book.

In *this* book, my aim is to help those who've had adverse medication reactions, complicated discontinuation syndromes, or withdrawals, whether it's from benzodiazepines, antibiotics, antidepressants, or any other medication that has left you mentally and physically compromised due to a central nervous system (CNS) injury. I hope this book will serve as a reminder to you and your loved ones that you have an iatrogenic CNS injury and need the time, love, patience, and support similar to someone who was injured in an automobile accident would and should receive.

I also hope this book can offer support to the people who love us, care for us, and who are trying to understand what the hell has happened to us. I want to offer a platform of validation for your experience and a few ideas that may be helpful as I share my trial-and-error experiences. In my roughest moments, it has been my hope that I could one day offer something of value to even just *one* person, which leads me to believe the pain and suffering will be worth it.

I hope you are that *one*. If not, thank you for reading, and I am so very sorry for what you are going through. At the very least, please know you are not alone.

"Every single person has a story that will break your heart. And if you're paying attention, many people… have a story that will bring you to your knees. Nobody rides for free."

- Brene Brown

I love this quote. "Nobody rides for free." It has helped me reframe this part of my life as my cost of admission. I pray that as time goes on, this part of the ride becomes less expensive. I also know I've had countless moments in my life when I gave no mind to what I had been granted, offered, and gifted without a worry of the cost. I am now aware. You cannot un-ring the bell, and I believe with all of my heart, mind, and soul that this process is like alchemy, and it will one day end and yield a more resilient, precious me. I can choose to look at this experience as a tragic test of my will, or I can open myself up to see it as an opportunity, albeit a painful one, that has the potential to be transformative on a bio-psycho-social-spiritual level. I want to pause here for a moment to reflect on what I just wrote. Do not get me wrong. I am not happy this has happened to me or to anyone else. Just as I am not happy about my loved one dying young of Alzheimers or losing friends and family to suicide, heart attack, cancer, and accidents. I have made a conscious decision to tell my story precisely because I think this particular health crisis could have been avoided had I been given proper informed consent. I know the level of suffering could have been minimized had there not been a second layer of gaslighting thrown on top of the heap. That said, just like in Brene's quote: "no one rides for free," while I believe this particular part of my journey could have been avoided, the cost of getting "stuck" in that sort of thinking will not help me, or anyone else. Advocacy and awareness can hopefully help others avoid this same potential pitfall. But, this book is based on a sense of "now what?" This is what I've got. It's the cards I've been dealt, fair or unfair, avoidable or not, and the attitude with which I choose to play this hand, I believe, can have a profound impact on how this journey unfolds for me.

Thanks for reading my story. I'll continue to share in future writing endeavors and on my blog on my website as my story evolves. It's important to tell yours, too. We all have a story to tell that needs to be heard. I'm listening.

A quick caveat before you proceed: *I am not a medically trained physician. What I speak about in this book are things that I found helpful/not helpful during my journey, and I am not offering prescriptive advice. One thing I have learned, and am continuing to learn on a daily basis, is that when it comes to our brains, our nervous systems, and our recovery to a medication injury, there isn't one answer that universally applies. This has been, by far, one of the most frustrating aspects of this experience. We can't go through this alone, and yet, in many ways, the only way we go through it IS alone. That said, this book is not designed to offer specific medical advice to serve as a substitute for receiving good clinical care. Benzodiazepine withdrawal can mimic many illnesses, mental and physical, and it is important that we do not overlook the possibility of other co-occurring illnesses or issues.*

As I continue to write, and as you continue to read, please know that all of what I will discuss are things I continue to strive to incorporate. Some days are much harder than others to manage and get through. It is a completely non-linear process of healing. There are many days that making my bed marks a "good day." Other days, I can try to participate in my life. It's so much easier on those good days to implement the strategies I will discuss that have been helpful. On the bad days, it is incredibly difficult to imagine doing any of them. Best of luck, I'm pulling for you!

CHAPTER FOUR

TRAUMA AND THE GRIEF PROCESS

"Trauma is personal. It does not disappear if it
is not validated. When it is ignored or invalidated
the silent screams continue internally heard only
by the one held captive. When someone enters the pain
and hears the screams healing can begin."

- Danielle Bernock

Trauma

Having worked with many clients dealing with various traumatic backgrounds, I was familiar with much of what constitutes and can accompany a trauma response. It was much easier being on the other side of the couch. Far easier than it was finding myself suddenly thrust into powerful fear and a sense of terror. Easier than experiencing ruminations that would lock me into myself for hours. And nothing could prepare me for the sensitivity and reaction to certain smells, sounds, and places that, consciously or unconsciously, reminded me of the health trauma I had experienced.

In explaining the concept of trauma to others in my clinical work, I had always shared that I believe it to be quite subjective, as well as having an enormous bandwidth in terms of what one might mean by *trauma*. I have always seen it as something that has basically *interrupted a process*.

"Trauma" is the Greek word for "wound." So, this wound, this interruption, this tear in the fabric of our expectations can encompass what some refer to as the *big T*: consisting of sexual, physical, or emotional abuse or neglect. However, traumas can also be losses of any kind—divorce, death, breakups, betrayals, loss of health, loss of job, bullying, being made to feel crazy or invisible, etc. Any events or changes that injure, wound, and tear at the fabric of our core sense of self and security. And while they may not be seen as traumatic by the masses, they can certainly be traumatic and, thus, need to be responded to as such. An experience of trauma is subjective based on that individual's sense of self and security. What is highly traumatic for one might not be felt that way by another. How one responds to the same event may be incredibly different than how someone else might respond.

There were a couple of traumas in my life prior to becoming ill that day in 2016. I lost my beloved grandmother a few months before my high school graduation. She died in a car accident, and her death tore me apart. It left me balancing on what felt like the edge of a cliff for years. I had wonderful parents, but my grandmother had been this quiet set of eyes that seemed solely designed to watch me with delight. She didn't say much, we didn't say much, but in her presence, I felt incredibly seen and cherished. I yearned for that quiet validation for nearly a decade after her death. If that validation dared to declare itself in a relationship, I would quickly sabotage it, as if allowing that need to be met was a betrayal to my grandmother and meant saying goodbye to her forever. It was through my own work on myself that I began to understand the trauma, the wound, the hole that her death had left in my sense of self and security.

Other traumas have included a few early childhood health issues, a dear family member's chronic and terminal illness, having friends pass away, and watching as people I loved battled addiction. I experienced my share of loss, but in many ways, during my first 46 years of life, my life was not riddled with trauma and grief. I hadn't had to face a health trauma that would leave me fighting for my existence.

Perhaps, in some ways, I wasn't prepared for the intense reaction I had towards becoming so ill, so fast. There are two constructs that I believe added to my struggle and made healing a bit more challenging. These are *second fear* and *secondary trauma*.

Second fear is a term coined by Dr. Claire Weekes in the 1960s in her international best seller, *Hope and Healing for your Nerves*. Dr. Weekes described an initial, automatic fear that is beyond our control, known as *first fear*. However, it was, she felt, *second fear* that was the problem for so many struggling with anxiety disorders. Second fear is the fear of fear. Fear of the state one is in or experiencing. This second fear perpetuates a fear-adrenaline-fear-adrenaline cycle that can lead one to feel like they are having a nervous breakdown of sorts and can lead to extreme nervous fatigue.

So, my experience of second fear went something like this: I would be unable to sleep and have strange thoughts that left me feeling disconnected from reality. I would then have a surge of adrenaline, but instead of returning to baseline, I would begin to fear that I would always feel disconnected, always feel strange. This fear kept the adrenaline surging, creating more symptoms, followed by more fear, followed by more adrenaline. You get my point. My fear of my state did not allow my already sensitized and compromised system a chance in Hades to calm down. Second fear is often accompanied by the thoughts, *What if?* or *Oh no!* It creates an attitude of fear that our uncomfortable thoughts, feelings, or bodily sensations will continue to appear, which almost always increases the likelihood for this to be the case. And as they reappear, our systems grow increasingly more sensitized, making the symptoms feel louder and scarier than before.

Anyone who has ever experienced a panic attack knows this pattern well. You are out shopping, begin to feel lightheaded, blurry vision, tunnel vision, palms sweaty and cold, your legs turn to jelly, and you fear you might pass out. You make it home, eventually calm, but the next time you need to return to that shopping mall, you're apprehensive, wondering, *What if that were to happen to me again*? Perhaps you can feel the surge of adrenaline, your heart begins to beat faster, and you feel jittery just in anticipation and in memory of what happened the last time. Many will manage this second fear by not returning to that shopping mall. In managing our fear and anxiety through avoidance, the world can quickly become quite small.

What I have learned from Dr. Weekes, and attempt to practice consistently, is her guidance to *notice* the feeling/sensation/ thought, *accept* that it is there (don't chase it down a rabbit hole or try to avoid it), *float* through it ("I feel this and know it's there, and I am going to float on through, and finish my shopping, my work, etc."), and then lastly, to *allow time to pass*. While this four-part sequence is very hard, the last one—*allowing time to pass*— is my nemesis. Apparently, I had been goofing off at the *virtue* banquet when they were handing out patience.

I'd like to take a moment and give a reverential nod to Dr. Claire Weekes. Both a PhD and an MD, Dr. Weekes led a seamless life between home and work (literally, she had patients come and stay in her home as she treated them for various nervous conditions). I believe her work some 60 years later is still the most straightforward, humanistic, and helpful source I have read or heard in understanding and treating anxiety. Her interest in working with people who grappled with anxiety stemmed from her own multi-year struggle with debilitating symptoms of anxiety—mainly unrelenting heart palpitations. Her symptoms were both misunderstood and misdiagnosed. She spent six months in a sanatorium being treated for tuberculosis that she *didn't have!* A year or two upon leaving the sanatorium, still struggling with chronic palpitations, a soldier who had been in war told her that it was her own fear that was causing and perpetuating the palpitations. This was her introduction to the mind-body connection and her theory of a sensitized system that can leave one ripe for developing all sorts of debilitating mental and physical issues. Dr. Weekes has, at times, received a bad rap as people have said she promoted the use of tranquilizers. However, if you listen to her television interviews, available on iTunes, you will see that even decades ago, she was only advocating for their use under the strict supervision of a doctor and for very brief periods of time. Please take the time to check out her books, her interviews, and her biography.

Even though I was a high functioning and mentally and physically healthy person prior to 2016, as well as during the years between what I deem "episode one" and "episode two," it is important to note this illness/injury during a bad moment or month has resulted in my meeting criteria for upwards of five to six DSM-5 diagnoses. The DSM-5 is the guide clinicians and psychiatrists use to diagnose individuals with psychiatric conditions. On a bad day I can meet criteria for anything from Major Depressive Disorder to Generalized Anxiety Disorder to Bipolar II, to OCD, to Borderline Personality Disorder. I decided to bring up this point while I am talking about Claire Weekes and "second fear" for a couple of reasons.

The first reason is I believe benzodiazepines are the next Opioid epidemic. However, unlike what has occurred with the Opioid epidemic, people who are struggling being on or coming off of benzodiazepines are not breaking into pharmacies, prostituting themselves, or committing other crimes in a desperate attempt to gain access to their medication/drug. We, instead, look like psychiatric patients. We find ourselves depressed, wildly anxious with all of its accordant symptoms (panic, intrusive thoughts, depersonalization and derealization, phobias, ruminations). Additionally, we are unable to sleep and may show a myriad of other mental and physical symptoms as our autonomic nervous systems are now unstable and unpredictable. People in benzo withdrawal are often labeled with the diagnoses I mentioned above as well as many others including, but not limited to conversion disorders, Bipolar Disorder, and Schizophrenia. I recently heard a statistic that nearly 80% of all benzodiazepines are NOT prescribed by psychiatrists and neurologists, those physicians with specific training in the brain and nervous system. Instead, this class of medication tends to be most prescribed by General Practitioners, Family Medicine doctors, Internal Medicine doctors, and OB-GYNs. Yet the myriad of symptoms their use and withdrawal often leave us with land us directly into psychiatrists offices and psych wards, often poly-drugged and now stuck on the hamster wheel of psychotropic medications in an attempt to manage our multitude of life-altering symptoms.

The second reason this is important is that even though I did not enter into taking the antibiotic or the benzodiazepine with anxiety, any other formal diagnoses, or an overly sensitized nervous system, I have all of the manifestations of them now. I can sit and simply wait for my brain and nervous system to heal. But I feel that waiting is not the only answer to this complicated mess we find ourselves in. Don't get me wrong, I strongly believe that TIME is an enormous factor in our healing. However, I have always believed that consistent effort plus time yields result. So, what do I mean by "effort?"

First, what that means for me is that regardless of WHY I now have all of these symptoms/reactions/sensations, I still need to look for the HOW in terms of navigating and responding to them. I don't want to simply *manage* my myriad of symptoms. I want to try to actively help myself and to attempt to effect change, if possible. Second, how I see effort has fundamentally changed for me. "Effort" does not always necessarily mean working harder, fighting more, being more persistent. I now see "effort" as including working smarter, focusing on a shift in attitude towards my symptoms and sensations, and slowing down to the speed of wisdom so that we are in a better position to see and generate other options. We get good at what we practice. So, let's practice "smart" things. For example, if I practice trying to lose weight by running more but my run consists of running from my bedroom to the kitchen 150 times a day to eat some peanut butter or ice cream, guess what happens? Sure, I get good at running, but I also gained 75 pounds! An example of "fighting harder" not necessarily equating to *smart effort* in our recovery can be seen in our response to all of the manifestations of anxiety we often endure in this process. With anxiety, less is often more. Letting go, floating, not engaging, leaving things alone, and adopting an attitude of "irrelevance" towards our anxiety is key. Anxiety feeds off our "fight" and our "working to get rid of" leads to it growing stronger and more pervasive.

So, for me, the idea of "second fear" was a place where I felt I could begin to work smarter and begin to effect change regarding many of my symptoms and my state of being. If I could practice not being so afraid of the state I was in, then at the very least I wouldn't be adding more fear, adrenaline, cortisol, and negativity to my already vulnerable experience and system. "Second fear" kept me very stuck for a very long time, and on my bad days, it absolutely creeps up and takes me under. But I continue to practice being mindful of this force of "second fear" and try to keep it in the forefront of my mind as I wake each day and make a decision as to where and how I will choose to expend my effort.

The other aspect that really kept me stuck was the *secondary trauma* I experienced, especially after my first episode back in 2016.

This secondary trauma was my being dismissed by so many in the medical community and being told that there was no way the antibiotic could be the cause of my symptoms. To compound this issue, years later, I received a similar response when I proved unable to come off the benzodiazepine without debilitating results. Having worked with many victims of rape, emotional abuse from narcissistic partners, and countless other traumatic histories, I was certainly familiar academically and intellectually with the concept of secondary trauma. I would help my clients find their way towards solid ground after years of gaslighting by their spouses, families, and the legal system. So, I knew something about it, but I had no firsthand, experiential knowledge of just how crazy-making, demoralizing, and destructive it could be to be disbelieved. This whole experience has led me to be a more empathic clinician and human being.

Another aspect of this secondary trauma was that the myriad of symptoms were mostly invisible or unmeasurable by clinicians, family members, and friends. The tremor in my spine, the forks and knives driving into my feet and legs, foggy goggle vision... no one could tell that anything above a *quiet, indoor voice* was over-whelming to me. They couldn't see the fear and terror that would come as the minutes ticked by, night after night, while trying to find sleep, and they could never know the impact of random, intrusive thoughts or a sudden sense of not being intact or even real. I had an invisible illness. I was always stunned when people would respond to me as if I was *normal*, when inside, I felt like an evil conductor had taken over most of my mental and bodily functions. This disconnect between how we feel and how others perceive us can add a layer of crazy-making to the experience.

My only option was to try to describe this litany of bizarre symptoms, but even well-meaning people had no idea how to help. And, quite frankly, I had no idea how or what anyone could do to help me. I thank God I at least knew I would first need to forgive myself and then begin figuring out how to get out of this deep hole.

Forgive myself? Yes, this is a huge part of the process and one I will go into further. I needed to forgive the doctor who prescribed me the antibiotic, forgive the medication, forgive the specialists who wrote me off, forgive the various people who didn't slow down to explain the potential for bad side effects. But to really heal, I had to forgive myself. I felt weak thinking, *Why am I one of those in the small percentage that have adverse reactions?* I found myself believing that I must have a weak constitution or that I was being punished for something. I had to stop that line of thinking before I could begin to really heal.

The Grief Process

Many of us are familiar with Elizabeth Kubler-Ross's five stages of grief: denial, anger, bargaining, depression, and acceptance. Brilliant is her summation of what we all face at various times in our lives. What's important to know is that these are not linear; you don't complete denial and move into anger. It's essential also to know that you can feel some more than others, some not at all, and you are swirling through any and all of them at the same time.

For me, the denial was really held by others. Again, I knew that I had been one way on a Friday morning, and 48 hours later, I was a different person. Thank God I had a strong enough sense of self to know that to be true and had many good friends and family who reflected back on who I had been, who I still was underneath this pile of pain.

Most of the denial, was ultimately mostly held in the eyes and words of others, as each symptom was written off and invalidated. I didn't want to be a medical mystery; I didn't want that kind of attention. I just wanted someone to say, "I don't know, but we are going to figure this out together." Initially, I did not have the literal brain power to sit and research neuro-toxicity or comb through the internet and medical journals in an attempt to grasp what happened. I just wanted to find some way to feel better, get back to my life, and forget the whole thing.

Once that wonderful ENT and my hairdresser confirmed for me what was occurring in my mind and body, I let go of what denial I was experiencing and was able to finally accept that what was happening was really happening and that there was a reason why. Also, having this information allowed me to not be so affected by the continued gaslighting I encountered as I was told my antibiotic reaction was everything from a "food allergy" to some sort of "conversion disorder." Once I was able to gain back a bit of my confidence, I moved out of denial into full awareness and began to work towards acceptance. I think this fact saved me in some ways. It allowed me from being com-pletely devoured by that secondary trauma. I knew it was real. I took an antibiotic, and it blew up my nervous system. What I didn't know was whether or not I would ever be the same.

This led to the bargaining, anger, and depression aspect of my grief process. Anger at myself for going to an urgent care center. *If only I had waited to see my internist maybe it would have been different.* Anger at the doctor and the pharmacist for not in-forming me that this was a very strong antibiotic. Anger at every specialist I talked to until that lovely ENT, who offered me a metaphorical, *I see you.* Anger at people around me going to concerts, out with loved ones, enjoying their lives. Anger at characters on TV who seemed well or could go to sleep at night. It seemed as if my anger was starting to take over, and the lens through which I used to see the world was lost. I was a victim. I was now just a stain and a burden.

This was all internal; this was my own process. I don't think anyone looking at me or engaging with me would have known how enraged and devalued I felt.

I also entered a time when I made all kinds of promises to myself and God. *If you just get me through this, I will eat only healthy. I will exercise more. I will take care of my body. I will go to church. I will be a better friend. I will help other people through this.*

Mixed in with all of this was a sinking feeling that my life would never be the same. That there was a *before* and an *after*. I was so sad, as I was not ready to let go of all that I had *before*.

In that in-between period of episodes one and two, I lived up to a few things I had promised in my *bargaining*. I did work on my faith. I did work on a life philosophy based on a study of Stoicism. I worked hard to pay attention to my overall health by limiting alcohol use, exercising, and eating (relatively) well.

During that first year or so, when I was focused on healing from the antibiotic injury, I experienced the luxury of actually getting better and trending towards health as the months went on. Strangely, some magical thinking went along with my bargaining at that time. I was making promises to God and myself, and I was getting better. As a result of this, I was spared (for a time) the depression many people experience when bargaining doesn't yield the result they are hoping to see.

It was very clear to me that no matter how much healing had occurred, I was not back to what I considered to be my baseline. I grieved the loss of clear vision; ears that didn't hum, buzz, or scream at me 24/7; and feet and legs that didn't prickle and burn. I was also aware that I became somewhat medication phobic. I was hypervigilant about not getting sick, as I was absolutely terrified of needing another antibiotic.

However, time lulled me back into my life, and as I said earlier, I didn't want to think back on how sick I had been. Whatever aspects of my grief I was *spared* in that first episode re-entered with a vengeance during my second episode.

As I awoke from surgery a few years later and realized all of the symptoms were back, albeit with less initial severity, I landed straight into depression. *No, this can't be happening again.* Over the next two months, as the medications I had previous success with seemed to be making me worse, I became too depressed to bargain. Days would slink by, and it would take all of my energy just to eat. Being able to bargain seemed to require an energy of hope, and on many days, I struggled to find my hope.

But as these symptoms would come and go, there were brief moments referred to as *windows* by Professor Heather Ashton. It was in these windows that I forced myself to get educated and started to do my own research. I found the *Ashton Manual,* written by Professor Heather Ashton out of the U.K., which seemed to be the only real guide regarding the misunderstood use of benzodiazepines and the need for a proper taper when discontinuing their use. I asked around, and no one had ever heard of it. I spoke to a few colleagues who ran rehabs and intensive outpatient programs for addiction. They, too, had never heard of it.

Once again, I found groups online and on Facebook for benzodiazepine withdrawal that had tens of thousands of members, with one group having over 90,000 members, all describing my exact symptoms. The stories of despair and trauma were often too overwhelming, but I began to realize, *Okay, this is a thing.*

I was no longer bargaining. I was starting to accept that not only had I been injured once by an antibiotic, but I had now been injured a second time. Information can be a friend and foe. At least it was for me in terms of accepting my situation. However, it was helpful to learn that a few key resources were out there for folks who had my symptom profile.

As much as all of this information about other people's experiences terrified me, it offered me the data to create a true plan and a sense that I didn't need to be okay with what had happened in order to radically accept it as my truth. Some of the best advice I have ever received was from my dad, who said, "The first thing you do when you realize you are in a hole is to STOP digging."

I recognized I was in a hellish hole. I thought I recovered from being *floxed* in 2016. I had woken up from surgery and appeared to have a resurgence of the original symptoms. I had gone back to my old stand-by medications to help me through it again. I realized they were not working this time. I had tried to come off the alprazolam, which most doctors de-prescribe by cutting the dose by 25% the first week or two, then another 25%, and continue with the assumption that most can *slide off* in a month or two. Remember, I got to a 30% reduction, and on day ten, the bottom fell out of my life. My hole was deep and seemed to get deeper and darker by the day. All of my energy went into the process of recognizing I was in a hole, trying to figure out how deep it really was, and how to get out of it.

Enter my new internist, psychiatrist, and therapist, along with a few key family members and friends. Their belief and support allowed me to string together moments of clarity and strength, put one foot in front of the other, live more often in the acceptance stage, and focus on managing my new reality.

This does not mean that I didn't or don't fall back into the grieving stages. Denial—*I can't believe this has happened.* Anger— *Why me? I am a good person. I don't do drugs. I take care of myself. This shouldn't have happened.* Bargaining—I do far less of this currently. Depression—this one comes up the most, especially in the mornings between 7:00 a.m. and 9:00 a.m. when the start of my day is filled with chemical anxiety, depression, and dread that is hard to put into words. But acceptance is where I try to live most of the time. Acceptance, gratitude, and a commitment to working a daily practice are key. Again, even as I write this, I am in a rough patch, and it can feel like gratitude and acceptance are unreachable. But I know that in an hour, a day, or a week, the clouds will part, and I will get a glimpse at just how much all of this daily effort and focus matters.

CHAPTER FIVE

AMOR FATI (LOVE/ACCEPT YOUR FATE)

"Nothing happens to anybody which
he is not fitted by nature to bear."

- Marcus Aurelius

It is fitting to write this chapter at the end of a day when the concept of *Amor Fati* was almost lost on me. One of the best things that has come out of this entire ordeal was my introduction to the philosophy of Stoicism. A younger brother sent me some information about this ancient philosophy years before, but I hadn't given it much thought.

In 2016, when I could finally read again, I skimmed a few books he recommended. With my foggy vision, it was often hard to read without a giant spotlight hitting my book in just the right way, but the concept of Amor Fati always stayed with me.

In my darkest moments, I found a gem in the writings and videos of Ryan Holiday. Do yourself a favor and look this guy up, read his books, subscribe to his free daily emails, and listen to his talks on YouTube. He is a young guy whose gift to take an ancient philosophy and apply it so aptly and clearly to our current lives and challenges is amazing.

What I came to learn and understand was that the principles of Stoicism were as relevant and applicable to the challenges of living in contemporary times as they were when Epictetus, Seneca, Marcus Aurelius, and others wrote them almost 2,000 years ago at the beginning of the Common Era.

When I run into the same messages in many different bottles, or when I encounter something hundreds (or thousands) of years old that resonates, I see this as stumbling upon a truth. Holiday, having learned the Nietzsche-coined concept of *Amor Fati* from author Robert Greene, felt that it captured a cornerstone and the essence of Stoic philosophy. Love your fate. I don't really think of it as truly loving my fate. Who can love losing a child, a loved one, or having an illness? I think of Amor Fati as a form of radical acceptance. Accept your fate and adopt the mindset to accept and make the best of your circumstances. Most of the time, we are not in control of what happens to us, but we are in control of our attitude and action toward those circumstances.

In fact, the very famous Serenity Prayer captures perfectly what I believe when I think of Amor Fati. *God grant me the serenity to accept the things I cannot change, the courage to change the things I can, and the wisdom to know the difference.* Health, balance, and resilience reside in these perfect words.

Let me accept the things I cannot change. I cannot change the fact that I took an antibiotic back in 2016. I cannot change the fact that the antibiotic injured my central nervous system. I cannot change the fact that I went on alprazolam and gabapentin to calm those symptoms, nor can I change the fact that I had a surgery that sent me back on those meds three years later. I cannot change the fact that I now have to endure a complicated withdrawal from these medications. For me, this is a tough one. The *what-ifs* and *if-onlys* can really take me under if I lose track and let myself start down the rabbit hole. It is hard to accept when bad things happen to us.

Another amazing book that helped me as I grappled with not becoming an injustice collector and focusing on *Why me?* was the book by the Buddhist writer Pema Chodron, called *When Things Fall Apart*.

Pema speaks about having a sign pinned to her wall that read, "Only to the extent that we expose ourselves over and over again to annihilation can that which is indestructible be found in us." She says that for her, it was all about "letting go of everything." Annihilation sounds like a dramatic and scary word. However, for those of you who have gone through being *floxed*, a benzo withdrawal, an antidepressant withdrawal, or a med injury, you probably know that our experience can often bring us to the brink of annihilation.

I have a dear friend who has helped thousands in their benzo withdrawal experience, and she states on one of her podcasts, "If someone who has gone through benzo withdrawal tells me that they haven't thought about suicide, I think they are lying." For me, and for many others, it isn't that we want to die or that we make a plan and are actively suicidal. It is simply the fact that there are times when you truly feel you cannot, and will not, survive this. That you cannot endure one more moment. I believe that is what Pema was speaking about in the brink of annihilation. And I believe that if we can get to that brink over and over again, and not go over the other side, we eventually will find what is truly indestructible about us and our spirit to survive.

Give me the courage to change the things I can. Little things I could change became important. My diet. I could control cutting out artificial sweeteners and sugar of any kind. I could abstain from alcohol and give up caffeine. These were a few things I could do that made a big difference. However, the most important way this showed up in my recovery process was the realization that the one thing that can never be taken from us is our attitude. So, what can I change? I can find the courage to change my attitude.

One way I did this was by thinking about all of the other people in the world right now suffering from physical, mental, and spiritual ailments. I would send prayers out to people I knew and many I didn't. Once in a while, I would get on GoFundMe and make a small donation to people I didn't know who were enduring something incredibly painful. I worked to be grateful and worked hard to recognize and remember that my attitude was the one thing that could not be taken from me. I began to slow down and think about how I was speaking to myself. I went from, *Oh no, what if I don't get better?* to, *Oh, I know I am going to get better.* I leaned on Wayne Dyer's play on words and instead of focusing on believing it when I see it, I started to focus on the knowing that I will see it when I believe it. Do not get me wrong. I was, and am, far from successfully mastering this practice. My attitude has made things much, much worse on many days, as I would slip into a state of fear, exhaustion, or feeling sorry for myself.

And the wisdom to know the difference. This is so key: practicing the act of slowing down and figuring out what is and is not in my control. This is a key principle in Stoicism. The wisdom to know the difference between what is and is not in one's control. On my most painful days, I found that my ability to slow down and gain this perspective would collapse. In the pain, the walls came in, and my view was myopic, urgent, and fear based. I needed to take what the Stoics refer to as a *view from the cosmos.* To stand high above and see our situation from a bird's eye view, a moment at a time. One moment in time to endure. And then the next.

Going back to my previous point about *second fear,* you can see how my challenge to radically accept my fate only perpetuated a trauma response of fear-adrenaline-fear-adrenaline-fear. Dr. Weekes and Stoic philosophers, as well as so many traditions in psychotherapy (CBT, DBT, ACT), stress the importance of right sizing our thoughts and using radical acceptance as a primary mode to regulate our emotions and tame our automatic trauma reactions.

For me, this is where I really turn to Claire Weekes, the folks in the DARE program (discussed in greater detail later), and also the work of Sally Winston and Martin Seif to guide me. Just like the title of this chapter, "Amor Fati," I believe a shift in attitude can greatly improve our recovery. Those of us with medication injuries, and especially those of us in benzodiazepine withdrawal, are experiencing a multitude of highly distressing physical and mental symptoms that are UNWANTED. What Weekes, DARE, and Winston/Seif discuss is that what needs to shift is our relationship with our distressing thoughts, fears, and physical sensations. Recovery isn't when you no longer have symptoms; it is when the symptoms no longer have you. However, secondary trauma is a major disadvantage for many of us. What we are experiencing has been simply written off as "not possible" and "not true." We can often be seen as feigning, malingering, or simply having a return of symptoms from a disorder we haven't addressed previously. What Dr. Sally Winston spoke about in an interview, and Claire Weekes spoke about decades ago, is that we need good information to then be able to implement the attitude of letting things be. For example, once Claire learned that it was her fear over her heart palpitations that kept them in place, she was able to practice floating and letting time pass. She took the magnifying glass off her heart wondering, *Oh no, what does this mean?* or *Oh no, what if this is going to kill me?*

For most of us we don't have doctors that are saying, "Okay, you have an iatrogenic injury from this medication that has led to an extremely raw and sensitized nervous system that has the potential to affect bodily functions, sensory functions, mental processing, your stress response cycle, and interplays with all of your other neurotransmitters, hormones, and chemical exchanges." If we did hear those words, then it would be more likely that when our heart missed beats or palpated; when we began to have racing thoughts; when we felt stuck in fight or flight; when we obsessed and then began to ruminate; when our skin burned, adrenaline surged, our ears whooshed; or our blood pressure plummeted, we wouldn't run screaming for the hills with "Oh my God!" or "Oh no!" or "What if?"

So, for me to begin my recovery, I had to do some research and come up with my confirmation of *This is what this is, Jen. You have an iatrogenic injury to your CNS, and it is highly sensitized and raw.* This has then allowed me to begin to adopt an attitude of allowance for these highly distressing symptoms. When I rush to Dr. Google or to the sites for the millionth time to type in a symptom, I try to gently remind myself that this is a form of "checking" and reassurance seeking that will give me short-term relief but ultimately lead me further down the rabbit hole.

Dr. Winston, in a recent DARE call, gave two great examples that I think are critical for us working to change our attitude and response to our situations. I will change them a bit to fit our unique circumstances. The first one: imagine you wake up in the morning and there is a new room in your house that magically appeared overnight. In that room is a giant mounted TV that is tuned into the "Withdrawal Station" where 24/7 there are scary thoughts, benzo lies of never getting better, weird bodily sensations, and loads of unwanted thoughts and feelings. There is no remote for this TV and you cannot figure out how to turn it off. It simply runs all day, every day. You can stay in that room staring at it and become overwhelmed. You can leave the room but go back in every few minutes to see if it is still there. Or you can leave the room, knowing it is still running, and allow it to be there while you go wash the dishes, go for a walk, read something interesting, or play with the dog. I don't know about you guys, but things get so overwhelming for me that I can spend all day every day throwing things at that TV trying to get it off the Withdrawal Station, and all I end up feeling is more frustrated and hopeless.

The second example was one Dr. Winston took from Acceptance and Commitment Therapy. Imagine you are throwing a very fancy, high-end party. You have spent tens of thousands of dollars on the event, including having fresh crab flown in from Alaska. In the middle of the party, you notice a man in bedraggled clothes, sort of smelly and grungy, standing at the buffet table eating some of the very expensive crab. You are getting more and more upset at his presence. He is ruining your party. All of your attention is now focused on this smelly intruder. Other people seem to notice him but are busy drinking, dancing, and socializing. But you are now completely obsessed with his presence and what to do about him. You have walked over and quietly asked him to leave, but he doesn't seem to hear you. Now you can either begin to yell and get irate or call the police to have him forcibly removed. Or you can choose to let him be, get engaged with the rest of your event and friends, and enjoy your party. I know what I would do and have done it a thousand times. I have begged my smelly intruder to leave. I have tried to pray him away. I have spent months focused on his presence and become so internally focused that the rest of my world and life have become nearly extinct. However, I believe if we can practice "Amor Fati" and shift our attitude from fight to float, it will not magically remove our withdrawal experience, our symptoms, or the smelly intruder, but in time, they will leave. In the meantime, we haven't added second fear to fear, we haven't become so internally preoccupied that we are making things worse, and we haven't been practicing being terrified of the state we are in. We have allowed our situation and all of its accordant unwanted symptoms to simply be.

During my recovery from these medications over the last six years, I have focused as best I can on this practice. Believe me, I am not great at it, and sometimes the chemical onslaught we face just makes a shift in attitude feel like a pipe dream. But we get good at what we practice.

While Ryan Holiday is not a doctor or a therapist, his books, *The Obstacle is the Way* and *Stillness is the Key*, and his *Daily Stoic* meditations speak to this allowing, accepting, and "smarter effort" mentality. These books became, and continue to be, important guides that provide a salve and remedy when hopelessness and despair descend.

Another of my favorite quotes is by Socrates: "The secret of change is to focus all of your energy not into fighting the old but building the new." Accepting the trauma, the interruption in the fabric of my old life, and learning to keep my eyes focused on the present is key. My darkest days are always intensified by looking back at what I used to be able to accomplish. I could work ten hours a day, run to see a friend, then run and grab a niece or nephew for a slumber party and not break a sweat. Now, any one of those things is difficult to achieve on a *good* day. The only way out is through, and we cannot look backward. How we *build the new* is by doing our very best every minute of every day. And sometimes doing our best simply means maintaining an attitude that we will see this painful moment, day, week, month, or year through, and we will undoubtedly be changed in the process.

Friedrich Nietzsche wrote, "He who has a why to live can bear almost any how." This quote is a bedrock for me in my healing process. There have been times when I spent hours holding tight to the *why* of my existence. I mentioned it at the beginning. Two words. *Aunt Jen*. Those two words are my *why*. Those words have given me more purpose, identity, pure love, and motivation than any other thing in my life. I became an aunt to Meghan at the age of 30 years. The best of me was born that year. This fall of 2021, I just welcomed my tenth niece/nephew. Aunt Jen is consistent, fun, available, interested, loving, goofy, hyper-vigilant about safety, and dedicated. These ten people offer me a platform to perform at my highest, most authentic level. This injury and process seek to rob me of these traits daily. Sometimes the injury wins. But I know that lurking underneath all of this is a new and improved Aunt Jen, and it is this thought that keeps my head above water during the harder moments. Find your *why*.

Viktor Frankl. This man and his work are life-changing. For those unfamiliar, get a copy of *Man's Search for Meaning*. Frankl spent years in a concentration camp while the rest of his family perished. Once released, he developed a psychospiritual therapy called Logotherapy that focuses on finding meaning in suffering. He writes about *attitudinal values* as being something that no one, and nothing, can strip away from us. They could take away his clothes, his food, and his loved ones, but they could not get inside him and take away his choice in how he would respond to himself. One of my all-time favorite Frankl quotes is, "Between stimulus and response lies a space. In that space lie our freedom and power to choose a response. In our response lies our growth and our freedom." This is a quote I fell in love with early in my career and have probably shared it hundreds of times with clients as I feel it is so powerful.

On days when the mental or physical pain feels unbearable, I search for this space between the stimulus (the pain) and the response. Many days I collapse that space, and my response is more of a reaction of self-pity, doubt that I could survive this, fear that I would never get better or only to get better to get worse again. But as I practice, and it does take LOTS of practice, I am able to see that I could still choose.

One of the things I have said to myself on my bad days (like today) is, *Even right now, as bad as you feel, there are tens of millions of people that would change places with you — this is bad, you feel awful, but there is still so much to be grateful for.* For those of you reading and thinking there could be no fresher hell than the one you are in, I know it feels that way. I always told my clients, "What is the worst kind of pain? It Is the pain YOU feel." We cannot know another's hell, no matter how empathic we are. So, how does one practice Amor Fati and come to fully accept their fate, when that fate is one of terrible pain? Practice. And for me, revisiting my faith.

CHAPTER SIX

FAITH

"Seeds of faith are always within us; sometimes it takes a crisis to nourish and encourage their growth."

- Susan L. Taylor

L et me start this chapter by being very clear that my intent is not to convert anyone nor to say that one faith path or belief is better than any other. While I am Christian, I have plenty of friends and clients who are Jewish, Muslim, Buddhist, Quaker, and many who are Agnostic or Atheist. But in telling my personal story of recovery, I would be incredibly remiss to leave this out as it has proven to be a game-changer for me.

I was raised in a home where my father had been reared Polish Catholic, and my mother was Baptist. For the first ten years of my life, they raised us as Christian. *Church* was our kitchen table where, on Sunday mornings, my brothers and I would take turns doing mini book reports on various Bible stories. I believed in God, but He was more like Santa Claus: a wonderful, fantastic idea. We were reared to see God as benevolent and kind, a protector. I will forever be grateful for that gift as I have worked clinically with so many people who were raised to see God as punishing and something to fear.

When I was ten years old, we moved to Houston, and my parents joined Memorial Drive United Methodist Church. That was now over 40 years ago, and this church still stands as the spiritual center for my mom and dad. My mom still volunteers by answering the phone every Wednesday, is on a funeral committee helping to serve at funerals, and helps with a book group. Every year, all of our stray pens would disappear for the *pen drive,* and our Sunday mornings would brighten through the inspirational words of Dr. Cragg, and our spirits would lift as the choir led us out with "Rejoice the Lord is King." Several of my siblings joined the church. I was married in it. However, after my divorce, I believe it became somewhat difficult for me to attend. Not because there was judgment; I never felt that. It was my own desire to find what God, religion, and spirituality would mean for me personally. It really wasn't until these last six years and this ordeal that my faith became my bedrock for all else in my life. I happened to find a wonderful church in Houston, which at the time, was led by a captivating minister named Howard Caesar. Howard has since left, but his successor, Michael Gott, is a brilliantly talented man who leads with humility and grace.

The best way I can describe how I see God was a description by who I believe was Neale Donald Walsh (please excuse me if I am attributing this to the wrong author). Probably 20 years ago, he visited and spoke at Unity Church of Christianity in Houston. The way I remember it was, he described God as like a mama in her large kitchen. Every morning after breakfast she would usher

her children into a large, fenced-in backyard. Out back all day, they could play, fight, create something, destroy something, build a garden, sit and do nothing, be resentful of their time in the yard, or be at peace with their day in the yard. They could make their time in the yard Heaven or Hell. At the end of the day, no matter how they spent their day in the yard, the mama would open the back door and call them all inside for dinner. This vision of God supported my youthful view of God as a helper, a non-judgmental protector. I am sure many Christians might think it's a very watered-down spiritual idea. But for me, it is what I believe, and it serves me.

It is this idea of the mama and the backyard that has always kept me present and focused on the fact that I was granted this particular time slot. The people around me, all of them, all of us here right now, are my neighbors. We were all granted this particular moment in time. What we do with it is up to us.

I had 46 years of good health, a good education, a strong family, and resources. I have had a blessed time slot. In the last six years, it can be very, very easy on a bad day to forget this fact. I believe we all have a dark night of the soul. A time when things are so tough, we can believe we have been forsaken. For some, it starts in childhood. For some, it lasts a week, but for others, it can be years. For many, it can be a lifetime.

For me, even in these tough many years, I can usually find one moment when I remember that I am going to be okay. Then I go back to my Stockdale Paradox of, *I will be okay. Today doesn't look to be that day, but one day I will, and for now, I have to get through this moment.* And when I can say those words, I thank God. I do not know why things must be so hard at times, but I do believe one day, it will all make some sort of sense, in some sort of timeline that is out of my control.

Again, I am not preaching how to think about God or even to think of God. I am simply sharing what I have come to rely on during this journey. It was easy to think about God as that loving mama when I was out in that backyard playing carefree, creating, loving, and soaking it all in. It has been far more challenging to feel like I'm getting the crap kicked out of me in that yard, and wondering why that mama isn't coming out to break up the fight and save me from the bashing.

After my second episode, I stumbled upon a wonderful writer and minister by the name of Max Lucado. His books, especially, *Anxious for Nothing,* were another literary go-to for me. He has an amazing talent of breaking down ideas and presenting them in a way that could reach a mind struggling to focus, and a pulse of faith, that would feel so faint at times, I wondered if it still was alive in me. I am very grateful for the comfort I found in Max Lucado's words and books.

I feel that faith has served as both the problem and the solution. It was a problem in the way I believed I was a person of faith, but it was not something I practiced nor relied on consistently. My relationship with God was not something I worked on or offered daily diligent attention and care. I believed that all of my caretaking was a way of serving God. I still believe that to be true. In my role as therapist, daughter, sister, aunt, and friend, I do believe that how I live is a way of serving God.

What I had always been lacking, however, was true care of myself. This precious bag of skin I was granted was the last thing I took care of. I confused being generous of spirit with believing I got whatever was left over, and, quite often, there wasn't much left. But in my particular faith—Christianity—I am instructed to love and trust God with all of my heart, body, mind, and soul. Since I view my life as a gift granted, then one way to show gratitude, love, and trust is by taking care of this mind, body, and soul. It is said to treat your neighbor as you would want to be treated. I was pretty good at this one, but self-care, self-love, and self-compassion took a backseat to most things in my life.

In deepening my faith, I now truly know that we have to care for ourselves first, so we can show up well for others. I believe my body kept score over the years. I remember when I got sick in 2016, I said, *God, just give me a couple more years. Let me see my oldest niece (a sophomore in high school at the time) off to college... just let me get there.* Be careful what you ask for... I did mostly heal from that time and was able to minimize the repercussion that first episode had on my family. And my niece did go off to college (go Irish!), and five months later, as I was opened up in surgery, so was my frazzled nervous system. I was no longer able to plow along or keep my symptoms somewhat under wraps. This go-round, my body and soul said, *It's time.*

It was time. It is time. Time to reshuffle the deck a bit and realize that my relationship with myself and God has to be healthy, intact, and vibrant in order to move through the rest of my life. As I said, I write these words in no way to convert anyone. I write to be seen and known and express my gratitude for realizing that stepping into my faith was critical. It was a beautiful life until it came crashing down, and I believe, with all of my heart and soul, that the next chapters will be exquisite, full, filled with grace and BALANCED.

CHAPTER SEVEN

MY TRAUMA TRIPLETS AND DEVELOPING YOUR VILLAGE

"The key is to keep company only with people who uplift you, whose presence calls forth your best."

- Epictetus

One of the most critical aspects of my recovery was figuring out who would be in my camp. While spending time looking up symptoms and reading people's stories of horror and pain eventually became too much for me, my recovery process was truly informed and had a fighting chance because of the internet-based forums and group chats. Through various Facebook groups, I realized that the antibiotic injury was not only a *real thing* but that it had a name, and thousands of people had similar struggles.

A few years later, when I realized I was in trouble and my brain would not allow me to come off the benzodiazepine in a common manner, I again found solace, comfort, and direction in Facebook groups as well as the online support group Benzo Buddies. It was only through these forums that I learned that many people needed to taper off slowly, and there was such a thing as micro-tapering. In that group, people were happy to help me find a taper-schedule that would work for me.

In one particular Facebook group, I made two friends and was introduced to a few others along the way. These two friends just happened to live relatively close by (one just outside of Houston, one in Dallas), and we became trauma triplets. Since first meeting them (one I've met in person, the other just by phone), there has not been one single day I have not checked in with them. Although our stories were somewhat different, we were a good match for each other. We all seemed to possess a strong desire to be off these meds, had not been on them for a long period of time, and had loved ones and families that were our top priority. In addition to my trauma triplets, I check in regularly with a few other people who have been off the medications for a while, and two women still tapering and struggling. They have all been pillars of support for me along the way.

One of my trauma triplets made a virtual introduction for me to meet Geraldine Burns, a benzo-veteran who had a horrific withdrawal experience, runs her own podcast, and works tirelessly to support, educate, and advocate regarding benzo awareness. If you have taken, take, or are thinking of taking a benzo (or are a clinician who prescribes these meds), please listen to her podcast called *Benzodiazepine Awareness*. Geraldine's story, her kindness, and her tireless accessibility to those that are struggling are incredible.

When things would become challenging, my trauma triplets, my other *benzo friends*, and Geraldine were my teammates.

Unfortunately, when I was going through my first episode with the antibiotic, I had been too scared to make any friends on the forums. I was simply focused on getting well and feared getting too involved would keep me stuck. In my second episode involving the benzodiazepine, I became painfully aware that I would need to find *my people* in order to survive. Although I had a wonderful clinical team and wonderful family support, I truly believe that unless you have gone through this, you simply cannot imagine the horrors that can accompany benzo withdrawal.

I think it would have been very helpful to have befriended a couple of people after being *floxed* as well. Loved ones and friends are well-meaning, but until you have experienced tendons spontaneously rupturing (one thing I didn't have, thank God), or screaming ears, or hot pokers playing whack-a-mole on your legs and feet, you cannot truly grasp what someone is going through.

I also experienced a struggle to connect with people from my *normal*, pre-injury world for a long period of time, and still do, even as I write this book. It's not because I don't love them, but because I feel an internal pressure to be the person they used to know—the confident, interested, calm friend, daughter, sister, or aunt. This is challenging because I often feel insecure, self-focused, and afraid of my own shadow. Feeling disconnected from those I love the most has been one of the most painful parts of this journey.

Over time, I have let myself off the hook of guilt and shame. I have come to see trying to maintain normalcy in life and relationships while navigating these symptoms is akin to having a picnic in a tornado. As much as I might want to see them, show up well, enjoy a meal or a conversation, and in essence, have that picnic, the storm inside of me can make it near impossible.

I also found it imperative to find my healing village outside of my family and non-medication injured friends because the process rendered me virtually unable to be reassured. I am sure many of you and your loved ones can relate. I had to realize this was not my fault, but I was driving people crazy nonetheless. Constantly asking, "Am I going to be okay?" or "What is happening to me?" and literally pummeling them with endless *what-ifs* and *if-onlys*.

I think about this *inability to be reassured* as a normal reaction to the *hell we didn't sign up for*. We weren't out smoking meth in an alley or going on the Dark Web to score loads of pills. I was, most of us were, simply taking medications as prescribed and trying to discontinue them as advised. I was doing everything right, or so I thought. So, how did it all take such a sharp turn and leave me in such an abysmal state? A state that progressed from mild discomfort to a full disintegration of myself. A total loss of confidence in myself, and the medical establishment, left me scouring for *anyone* to tell me I was going to be okay. But when anyone uses reassurance in an effort to alleviate a distressing feeling or sensation, the relief felt is only temporary at best, and more often than not, ends up making things worse.

It's like skydiving. One person signs up, has always wanted to do it, researched it, found the best and safest service to use, can't wait for the big day, and as they jump out, they are smiling and enjoying the adrenaline rush all the way down. Then there's the person who was told they were just going for a leisurely airplane ride. Even though they forced on two parachutes, have grabbed three more on the way out, and have been ensured they will be fine as they are tossed from the plane, they are screaming the whole way down, "Holy shit, am I going to die!? Someone, anyone, help me!" I am the latter. Most of us going through this are. Checking and re-checking our parachutes, nothing really quelling our terror, and screaming, "Get me off this ride!" Unless you have been through it, it's hard to understand why we need to ask the same damn question, day after day, sometimes all day long.

So, regardless of what medication you have been injured from—whether it is an antibiotic, antidepressant, a benzodiazepine dependency, or any other adverse response to a medication—do yourself a favor and find your village.

Once I found this village, it became very necessary at times to take breaks from the sites and boards. This is much easier said than done and not something I am good at maintaining. I was too vulnerable, and learning about the pain and suffering of others was overwhelming. I found myself suddenly spending hours looking up the latest random symptom I was experiencing. I had to remember, *Get back to my people.*

Having my village makes it so I don't have to share my story or struggle with friends and family along the way. Sure, I keep them informed, but having my team helps ensure all my other relationships don't center around what I go through every day.

I can honestly say the bonds I have created with my triplets, a couple of others along the way, and Geraldine are amongst the most precious and vital in my life. They have, and continue to, save me in unimaginable ways. Also, having my parents, therapist, best friend, and family behind me keeps me alive. Literally. I realize in typing those words just how lucky I am. I have met so many that lost loved ones because the strain of the chronic, invisible illness was just too overwhelming, or they just couldn't believe that a medication could leave one in this condition. I didn't have the secondary trauma of losing my friends and family like so many others have endured. I am eternally grateful to have a family behind me who was curious enough to read articles, look at YouTube videos, listen to podcasts, and learn how to be helpful. For those of you that don't, it is even more imperative that you find someone to walk with through this process. In his interview on *The Inner Compass Initiative*, Chris Paige states that he lost nearly everyone and everything. He met a couple of people online on the support sites who were his lifeline and continue to be his best friends to this day.

So, reach out and find a friend or two. Get a trauma twin, triplet, or a small village to keep by your side. Along the way, I have been a support, as well as been supported, which has made all the difference.

CHAPTER EIGHT

MENTALOMICS

"The universe is full of noise. True wisdom is in knowing what to pay attention to."

- Debasish Mridha

"Mentalomics" is a term I came up with and have used in my clinical practice for years. I use it to describe the notion that we do not have infinite psychic energy, and thus, we have to be quite discerning about where we choose to put our attention. It was in my study of Freud back in graduate school that I read about his economic theory. In essence, Freud was referring to our flow of libidinal energy (life force, sexual, creative energy) that flows through us as we navigate various life tasks and developmental phases. He would describe that if a trauma occurred as we traversed through our psychosexual stages (oral, anal, genital, latency, adolescence), that energy could get trapped there, and we would need to find a way (from his perspective, psychoanalysis) to unclog the trauma at its source to avoid becoming fixated and stuck along the way. In other words, if we start with a hundred units of energy to get us through our lives successfully, but we encounter major traumas (interruptions) along the way, co-opting that energy, we will have less and less to sustain us on our journey of development.

For me, this idea really began to make sense years later. I had been working as a therapist for well over a decade and was home ill one day. The kind of ill where you don't even have the energy to change the channel. So, there I lay, and the show "The Deadliest Catch" was on, and it was a marathon. I had never seen the show before, let alone watched 11 episodes back-to-back. Dozing in and out, dazed, and drenched in fever, I watched and watched as various crews took their boats out into the giant, freezing Bering Sea to catch crabs. About eight hours in, I sat up on my couch and grabbed a notebook. I began to quickly and feverishly (literally) write out what felt profound to me. Suddenly, Freud's theory made sense to me on a deeper level.

I watched as these various crews would head out to sea for weeks at a time in hunt of a certain type of crab. They weren't looking for fish, lobsters, or anything else—just crab and a particular size of crab to boot. The large waves rocked their boats, and it seemed like cold and dangerous work. They would release enormous cages, they referred to as pots, into the sea, and mark them with giant buoys. Many hours later, they would return to pull up the pots and dump them onto a huge sorting table, like a child dumping their Halloween bags, excited to see their new treasures. But what fascinated me about this process was how efficient and effective they were at discerning what they should keep and what they should not. As they pulled these enormous pots onto their boats and dumped them out, men in bright yellow slickers began quickly sifting through the fish, starfish, and sea debris to quickly get rid of everything that did not fit their goal. There were even crabs that made it on board that made the quick toss off, as they were not the right type or size. The rest were quickly tossed into a holding tank below deck, and then off they went again in search of the next pot to pull.

As I watched, I thought, *This is such a metaphor for our minds and living effectively.* These guys knew what they were looking for. They didn't stand around holding up a starfish, saying, "You aren't what I wanted! What are you doing on my boat? Why are you here? Why can't you be a crab?" No, they simply identified that this is not what I am looking for, and all the begging in the world would never transform that starfish into a crab, and they let it go and continued to focus on what would serve them.

So much of our lives are focused on the negative things that cross our paths, land in our lanes, or jump on our boat. Focusing on them deters or delays us from focusing on what is good for us and what will bring us closer to our goals. Why did that person just cut me off in traffic? Why didn't my boss appreciate my extra effort? Why did I get sick or injured? Why was that person rude to me?

Imagine that fisherman standing on deck of his crab boat, holding up a starfish, and instead of quickly recognizing it is not what he needs and tossing it overboard, he stares at it, getting more and more upset, thinking, *Why did you go into that pot? You aren't a crab.* As he paces back and forth, willing that starfish to be a crab rather than what it is, he becomes increasingly more upset. It's a starfish, and it will never be a crab. When he finally tosses it off, he finds himself unable to move on and is focused on feeling defeated, deflated, bothered, and thinks, *What the hell? That isn't how this is supposed to go—I am here to get crab.*

We have to know our *intention* so we can be better at recognizing and not spending time on what we need to let go of. This doesn't mean that surprises can't land on our boats that may be better for us than our original goal. So, some flexibility and discernment are absolutely required. But my point is that we often spend far more energy on, *Why me?* rather than, *Why not me?* So, toss the starfish to the side and keep moving.

My medication injury was my giant starfish. It came on board my boat—my boat that I believed was headed for lovely shores and a wonderful bounty of crab—and stopped me in my tracks. It's six years later, and as various symptoms continue to rear their head, I can get *very* stuck thinking, *Oh no, what is this?* I can lose hours, sometimes days, researching, looking up who else might have this symptom, and then comparing myself with others. I can also lose hours and days feeling down, despondent, and thinking, *This shouldn't be happening to me.* But it is happening to me. And I often have to work hard to remember to *toss the starfish! It is never going to be anything other than what it is, and you can't afford to ponder and try to change it.*

I don't have endless psychic energy. I can't expect to live a calm, grounded, focused life if the turds in the road, or starfish on my crab boat, stop me in my tracks. I can slow down, see if there is some way it can serve me, make an efficient decision to adapt, to let it go, or move in a different direction. However, with my brain and nervous system being in such a limbic loop of fight, flight, or freeze, it has not been as simple as *just accept the starfish and throw it back into the sea* or *see the turd in the road and just step around it*. It's not that simple. Sometimes the symptoms are just too debilitating. I have found it requires a conscious, daily practice to gain the skill set of accepting and allowing my new reality while not getting stuck and paralyzed in the analysis of it. Simultaneously, I must continue working to keep my sense of self intact, with my goals and values guiding me to let go of the *Why me?* mentality. This mentality is a waste of precious energy. The *Why me?* has a place in our grief process, but in the economy of our mind, it is akin to the Boardwalk property in Monopoly; it's very expensive. The *Why me?* will never yield a house or hotel. The only monopoly it will ever earn is one of getting on the nerves of everyone you love, including yourself!

This is another example where our injured minds are just like everyone else's. Every person, healthy or sick, makes cost/benefit analyses on an hour-to-hour basis, without noticing. *If I eat this piece of cheesecake, I may need to work out 15 more minutes.* Or, *If I decide to fight this fight, I will be exhausted but I need to stand up for what I believe in.* Or, *if I decide to drink tonight, I may feel unwell tomorrow, and I have that baby shower at 2:00 p.m.*

All day long, folks make decisions using a cost/benefit analysis: Mentalomics. For us injured folks, it's the same. On a less symptomatic day, I may feel like I can walk an extra mile or eat off of my rigid dietary plan, but I have to do so knowing I will likely pay the piper at some point in the future.

I have found that, since injured, my reactions are delayed. I can get on the phone and help a friend go through a difficult moment and feel just fine while I do it. Then a day or two later, I will feel symptomatic and struggle. It has taken me a while to recognize this pattern that my nervous system doesn't seem to respond to stressors in real time. Now that I know my pattern of response, I use that data to decide what to invest my time and energy in, knowing that I may face a very distressing, albeit slightly delayed, reaction. This has actually proven to create a positive change in my life. I have been going through my withdrawal during a time of great political divide, and in the midst of a pandemic, with which there has been great debate regarding issues such as the vaccine and social distancing. It didn't take me long to realize that if I engage in any sort of heated dialogue about politics, the pandemic, or other *hot* topics, I can spend upwards of a week trying to wind down and managing symptoms, such as feeling my brain and spine literally burn, screaming ears, and shooting pains in my legs and feet.

A dear friend of mine, also managing a challenging withdrawal from a benzodiazepine, was "kicking ass" in managing a very complicated and highly conflictual situation in her life. But just a week later, she called crying, feeling overwhelmed, depressed, and non-functional. As we traced it back, we realized she was simply paying for what had happened the week before. For many non-injured folks, they tend to feel the stress as it is happening or soon after, so their mental and physical reactions make sense to them, as they are feeling their stress response in relative real time. They feel overwhelmed during overwhelming circumstances. For me, I realized I was, and always had been, pretty good at crisis management, but in my injured state, I would pay dearly a few days later. I felt demoralized and confused until I recognized the pattern. Even in recovery, we do have to tend to life, and there are certainly times the consequence of an increase in symptoms is worth it. However, it's important to choose wisely where we place our very precious and valuable time, attention, and energy.

CHAPTER NINE

INTENTION, ATTENTION, AND REFLECTION

"What you do with your attention
is in the end what you do with your life."

- John Green

M y first job after graduate school was in hospice care. During my first month, I was taught the profound process of intention, attention, and reflection. While the woman who taught this to me did not use these words, they are, in essence, what she described. It was an overwhelming job, and from day one, I felt I was in over my head. Sitting with the dying was not something I could sustain for long, or so I felt. I felt I needed to leave and handed in my two-week notice to my boss. She was shocked and asked why I felt the need to leave so abruptly. I explained that it was overwhelming, I was in over my head, the work was intense, my case load was high, and I felt like I was running around like a chicken with its head cut off. She handed me back my resignation letter and asked me to give her two weeks. "Two weeks," she said, "and at the end of it, no need for a notice. You can just walk out." With nothing to lose, as I had already planned on being around for two more weeks, I agreed. She told me to take the next day off and return to the office on Monday at 8:00 a.m. and to report directly to her office.

When I arrived on Monday, she asked me to walk her through my process. I had no idea what she meant. She asked, "What does your daily routine look like?" I didn't really have one. It was the days before cell phones, and the area I covered was all of central Houston, all the way out 50 miles north and 30 miles east. In one day, I could spend three to four hours in my Jeep, driving from one home to another. No Mapquest, no cell phone, just a pocket full of quarters for pay phones, an orange key map book, and my nifty pager that sent messages like, "Dave P just passed away in Baytown family needs you," instructing me to turn around, and head across town.

My boss asked me to begin each day by spending 30-45 minutes mapping out my day to the best of my ability, literally and figuratively. Then she instructed me to get in my Jeep, turn the AC on full blast. (I drove a soft top Jeep, and it could be well over a 100 degrees with the heat index in summer.) While I was waiting for my Jeep to cool, she told me to look at the face sheet of the first person I would be visiting. The face sheet is the form that holds all identifying information—name, age, diagnosis, family members, etc. She taught me to say their name out loud, to think about if this was a first-time visit, or someone I had seen before, and if the latter, to reflect on our last meeting. She was asking me to be *intentional* about what I was doing. Then as I drove to their home, I was to turn off all music about five minutes before arriving and take a look around, take in the neighborhood, the environment, and mindfully observe my surroundings. Then, as I pulled up in front of my patient's home, and before I turned off my Jeep and the lovely AC, I was to once again look at the face sheet and say the person's name out loud. She instructed me to look at the family members' names, so that I might be prepared for who might be greeting me on the other side of the door.

Being intentional, she taught me, made it much more possible to offer my full *attention* once I rang that bell. I wasn't thinking about music. My mind hadn't drifted. I wasn't thinking about the last patient or the next one. I was present. Once my visit was complete, I was to turn on my Jeep, and while I let it cool off, I was to say the patient's name again and *reflect* on what had just occurred. How had the meeting gone? Who had been there? Was there anything I needed to take care of for them once back at the office? Then, and only then, once I had fully closed my experience with this person, was I to take out the next face sheet and key map and spend a moment opening myself to the next experience.

This technique of opening and closing, and thus, focusing on intention, attention, and reflection is my favorite form of mindfulness. It is one that allowed me to remain working with the dying for many more years. It has served me solidly throughout my career and in my personal life when I *remember* to implement it. I have taught this process to many of my patients, but I always share that this requires a lot of practice. We get good at what we practice, but even now, over 25 years later, it is something that I forget to do often, and it takes very little for life to feel overwhelming.

In my recovery, I practice multiple times a day to remember this process. On a good day, it is easier to implement. On a difficult day, it is so challenging to both remember and implement it. However, slowing down to the speed of wisdom and meeting my moment, my hour, my day with intention, attention, and reflection makes all the difference in the world. I can open the morning and close the evening, having made it through a difficult day. I can open and close a bad hour and not let my monkey mind run off thinking I will feel like this forever. Try it. It's magical. But remember, it's a practice, and although we get good at what we practice, I have never found that this practice becomes habitual. I have to consciously work at it each and every time.

CHAPTER TEN

SLOWING DOWN
TO THE SPEED OF WISDOM

*"Sometimes I think there are only two instructions
we need to follow to develop and deepen our
spiritual life: slow down and let go."*

- Oriah Mountain Dreamer

Helping people slow down to the speed of wisdom is a construct I have used in my clinical practice with clients for a long time. When we are uncomfortable, in distress, panicked, or in pain, it is natural to want to *get out* of that state as quickly as possible. Unfortunately, through healing from antibiotic toxicity and going through benzodiazepine withdrawal, I have learned that slow and steady wins the race. It doesn't mean it's comfortable. In fact, one of the first pieces of advice I was given in this process was, "Get comfortable with discomfort."

During this process, I have made a ton of mistakes. Many were because I wanted a quick answer to manage any number of symptoms that might pop up. I wanted to taper off the meds faster—a huge mistake. I wanted to add something in or take something out, and I would often make too many changes at once and then have no idea what was causing each reaction.

A word of caution: if you are going to add in or remove anything (a food, supplement, medication, etc.), do it slow and steady and one at a time so you can actually track what is creating each reaction. If you add in or remove too many things at once, you will have too many variables to consider, and it can become incredibly confusing and overwhelming.

There is nothing about the world we live in today that helps us slow down. Everything is instant and fast. Our food, our groceries, our communication, our deliveries. We get frustrated if our Amazon deliveries don't arrive in 48 hours or our groceries aren't at our door in two hours as ordered. There is no other process that will teach patience like that of withdrawal, discontinuation from medications, and having adverse reactions, in which time is your greatest and often only ally. It's painful to go slow.

My dear friend Dr. Blake Haren, a psychiatrist in Tennessee, frequently reminds me to slow down and be kind to myself. On a particularly bad day, I reached out, and he said, "Jen, you have to take extra precautions to protect yourself during this process. Things like guilt, shame, and not being kind to yourself are going to interrupt your healing. You have to slow down and allow space for curiosity and self-compassion, so you can better understand this injury and assess what is helpful and what is not."

In an interview with Chris Paige on the *Inner Compass* Facebook site, he describes his nearly four-year process of torturous, daily akathisia following a rapid benzodiazepine detox in a medical detox facility. In that interview, he painfully explains that there was nothing he could do besides "trust the process." Had he quit at the three-and-a-half-year mark, he would never have known that in just a few short months, he would be improving and moving out of his hell. There have been times in this process when each minute can feel like an hour. But there is no way out but through. I have found slow and steady is the only way to do it.

CHAPTER ELEVEN

WHAT A DIFFERENCE A DAY MAKES

*"In three words, I can sum up everything
I've learned about life: It goes on."*

- Robert Frost

What a difference a day makes. I cannot tell you how many times in my recovery processes (both of them) I would sing or say this phrase to myself. At one point, I took my own clinical advice, and on a pretty good day following a very scary episode, I wrote myself a letter. A letter to *bad day me* from *good day me.* If you have gone through a medication injury, you will understand perfectly what I mean. *Bad day me,* prior to becoming ill, was moody, upset, or maybe sad. *Bad day me,* after having been floxed and benzo poisoned, wasn't sure I wanted to live. It's hard for me to admit that aloud, even to myself. I certainly hate that my loved ones, especially the kiddos in my family, will read this, but it is absolutely true. There have been bad days, or weeks, that were so black and void of any virtue or truth that I was uncertain that I had the strength to last more than a few more moments.

So, it always surprised me when parts of me would rise out of the ashes either later that day, later that week, or sometimes even later that month. I could literally feel the clouds part, and as I stepped tentatively towards the light, fearing my own fragility, I would tell myself, *Don't forget how bad that was, and don't forget, you always come out of it.* However, each and every time, I would do just that. I would start to feel *normal* and forget what the blackness felt like. Unfortunately, it was because of the situational amnesia (a choice I was making, to push it away) that I would plunge back into despair each time the floor beneath me gave way.

It was very helpful to write that letter to myself. Right there, in black and white, a reminder that things can and do get better if we just *let more time pass,* in the words of the aforementioned Dr. Claire Weekes. So, we can likely agree that the term *bad day* means a whole different level of hell than anything we knew in our pre-injured state. Do yourself a favor; the next time you come out of a tough moment, immediately write yourself a compassionate letter, reminding yourself not to get hooked by the thought you will be stuck in that moment forever. Let a little more time pass.

CHAPTER TWELVE

BE LIKE PENNY

"When we are no longer able to change a situation,
we are challenged to change ourselves."

-Viktor Frankl

One of my mom's closest friends is a woman named Penny. When I was about 11 years old, I met Penny when her family moved into our Houston suburban neighborhood. My mom, always the caretaker, heard that a woman moved into the neighborhood from Oklahoma due to her need for a heart transplant. She was 38 years old, married with two small kids, and had lost her oldest daughter, who was my age, to a similar heart issue just a couple of years before. My mom reached out to Penny, and to this day (yes, Penny is still alive nearly 40 years after having a heart transplant), they are the closest of friends. Penny survived the death of a child. A loss I could not begin to imagine. Then she had to face her own potential death, a risky procedure, an even riskier life with a transplanted heart, and a host of, "We will just have to see," in response to her questions of whether or not she would be okay. What I remember about Penny was that she did recover, she bought herself a Porsche, and she resumed her work as a speech therapist. I was too young to really grasp what an incredibly strong woman she was. I was too young to understand living with grief and uncertainty of your own future. I didn't understand just how brave it is to face the unknown and truly live and love fully.

However, in my journey of this medication injury and my own uncertainty, I now see what an amazing spirit it requires to do what Penny did, and continues to do, daily. There have been more times than I can count when I have felt the piercing unfairness creep into my mind and send me reeling into self-pity and a darkness that scared me. I would summon up the image of Penny in my mind. I would sometimes use *Be like Penny* as my mantra. If she could lose a child and survive, if she could almost lose her own life, if she could live each day unsure if this new heart would continue to beat... then, surely, I could survive this too.

It's important to remember, though, that the worst kind of pain is your own. So, in my darker moments, this summoning of Penny did not always work. What I have learned about how I process the mental and physical duress that comes with my particular injury is that I can quickly become myopic. Meaning there are times I cannot see behind, around, above, or below my particular distress in certain moments. It is at those times that I feel most lost. This is when I have to just let more time pass, pray, and rely on my faith to kick in. This is when I also call on my beloved grandma to watch over me—to just let me ride out whatever particularly nasty wave of symptoms has washed over me.

That said, *Be like Penny* has helped me through some incredibly tough moments. I find it helpful to look at survivor stories. People I know, people I don't know. Our will is stronger than we can imagine. Thank you, Penny, for providing me with a model of resilience and strength. Find your Penny. They can serve as a beacon of light in the fog of our injury.

Since writing this chapter, sadly, Penny has passed away. On the morning of May 25, 2021, the world lost a beloved soldier. Rest in peace, Penny, and thank you for your lesson.

Chapter Thirteen

Little Signs Along the Way

"There are no accidents… there is only some purpose that we haven't yet understood."

- Deepak Chopra

We may agree to disagree on what I am about to share. I wouldn't want it any other way. I believe in discourse, and I believe there is plenty of room at the table for various opinions, thoughts, ideas, and experiences. Well before any of this ever happened to me, I believed in something larger than me, guiding me. I have always respected the idea that I am a part of something much larger and more complicated than I could grasp. This idea came through periodic *signs* I would receive that seemed to communicate to me that I was on the right path and was going to be okay.

This began about 18 months after my grandma had been killed in a car accident during my senior year of high school. I was off at college in San Marcos, Texas, and there was a guy who lived in the apartment downstairs who I felt might have a crush on me. I was seriously dating a big, handsome football player from another school and had no interest in thinking about anyone else. This guy from downstairs, let's call him Brian, would wait for me at the end of the street as we both had a statistics class together. Then it became clear he memorized my schedule and was always just kind of showing up. He was kind and shy.

One day, he saw my boyfriend, and I remember feeling my heart tug, when all 5′ 2″ of him said, "Was that giant dude your boyfriend?"

I laughed and said, "Yep."

He never came on to me, but he was simply always just there, walking me to and from class. We never spoke much except about statistics. I didn't even know his last name.

As we walked back to our apartment complex after completing our final exam, he asked if he could come up to my apartment. I found this bold, and must have had a strange look on my face, as he said, "No, it's just there's something I need to give you." You can imagine I found this comment to be strange, but I felt compelled to agree for some reason.

I remember he came into my bedroom, looked around, and said, "Okay, here it is." He held out a tape cassette (it was 1989) and said, "Play the third song, and I'll be back later." He left, and I put the tape in and forwarded it to the third song. The song was "He Walked On Water," by Randy Travis. Ten seconds into the song, I was in tears. It wasn't about a grandma, but suddenly, and immediately, it opened the floodgates that I had been holding sandbags against to keep the grief of her death at bay. *She walked on water in my mind* was a phrase I used to describe my relationship with my grandma to the one or two people I opened up to about her. As I played the song a third time, covered in snot, and with eyes so swollen, I couldn't see, Brian walked in, and hugged me. All he said was, "I was supposed to play that for you." We didn't speak. He held me until I fell asleep. When I woke up, there was a note that said, "The tape is for you—you will be okay." I never saw Brian again.

A similar experience happened a second time, about six years later. I had graduated with my Master's Degree in Social Work from University of Houston, and I had started my first job working as a Hospice Social Worker. I would travel to the homes of the dying and offer support and counsel to them and their loved ones. As I said before, there were many times I simply felt like I was in way over my head. I always feared death. Now, I was the one trying to help folks face it? What had I done? I was overwhelmed, depressed, and felt like a fraud. One night, I was in the office late, working on paperwork. I began to cry and found myself on my knees for the first time in my life. I don't know if I spoke out loud, but I remember saying, *Grandma, please tell me what to do… how can I help people when I don't even know what happened to you, where you are, if I will ever see you again? Are you underground or are you with God? How can I sit with anyone and comfort them when I have no idea what I believe?*

I stayed down on my knees for quite a while before I realized it had grown very dark outside; it seemed there was a storm blowing in. By the time I walked out to my car, it was incredibly windy, whipping my long hair into my face and blowing the stack of papers nearly out of my hands. As I approached my car, I noticed something was lying on the ground directly in front of the driver's side door. It was a small paper package, and surprisingly, it wasn't blowing away. As I got closer, I bent down to pick it up, my hair still whipping around my face and head. It was an empty pack of Pall Mall cigarettes in the maroon package—the very kind my grandma smoked until the day she died. There was no smell to the package, not a trace of tobacco, and yet that empty vessel had laid there amidst 20-mile-per-hour winds, and waited for me. It was that moment of knowing. There could not have been a clearer sign. I continued to work with the dying for another nine years.

Fast forward to Spring of 2020, when I am a month or so into the second episode of my struggle and having a particularly tough time. I am lost, alone, and terrified. I asked my grandma to please lead me through this. To show me how to heal. I begged her and God to help me find my way and to feel better. Within a week, I was ten times worse. This was not the answer I had been hoping for, nor expecting. As the bottom came out of my world that March, I was angry, sad, and beyond scared. But there was some small part of me that thought, *Is this going to get worse before I can get better? Is this healing?* Then, over the next few months, I found a support group online, made a couple of friends going through the same thing, and began to gain information about how to taper myself off of these medications safely.

A few months later, I was having a particularly bad day. I felt hopeless and despondent. The chemical depression and anxiety that accompany withdrawal were heavy and relentless. I again asked, *Grandma, where are you*? A couple of hours later, my best friend, who was with me at my folk's lake house, and helping me during a particularly rough patch in my recovery, called from an errand she was running. She said, "Jen, you aren't going to believe this… I'll be home in 15 minutes!" When she got back to the house, she ran to my room and showed me an empty, maroon-colored box of Pall Mall cigarettes just like what I had found 25 years earlier. She had been praying for me, and as she was walking to her car, she saw this lying on the ground. I started to cry, and told her that in a moment of panic, I called out to my grandmother. While I didn't feel an immediate lift from my physical and mental symptoms that day, I was reminded that I was not alone. Something larger was at play.

Then, around Christmas of 2020, I hit another really rough patch halfway through my turtle-speed benzo-taper. I was feeling adrift again, and my symptoms were mounting and scaring me. As I often did, I reached out to my friend, Geraldine Burns, and she kept reassuring me to just hold on, let time pass. I prayed to my God and my Grandma again, and said, *Please show me I am going to heal, please tell me I am on the right track.* I decided to listen to one of Geraldine's podcasts, as my eyes were too blurry to read or watch TV. I winced as I listened to Geraldine interview a young woman describe an utterly hellish experience coming off benzos. Her husband abandoned her, and she was left to rear her three-year-old daughter while completely incapacitated by the withdrawal. As Geraldine wrapped up the interview, she asked the young woman what she would want to share with other people going through withdrawal. The young woman said, "I want to end with a quote." Before she said another word, I felt goosebumps erupt all over my body. The voice of this woman I did not know quoted my all-time favorite quote, "Between stimulus and response lies a space. In that space lie our freedom and power to choose a response. In our response lies our growth and our freedom." I once again began to weep.

I do believe we are not alone in this. I do believe we heal. I do believe there are signs along the way. I do believe we can find hope in a newfound friend, in a trauma twin or triplet, and in the glimpses of health and wellness we get along the way. I am forever grateful for these signs. I have to believe that in the deep fog and storm, they are my guideposts that say, *this way,* or *just a few more miles to go.*

Chapter Fourteen

Building Back Your Confidence

"Confidence is contagious. So is lack of confidence."

- Vince Lombardi

D r. Claire Weekes spoke about a need to practice rebuilding our confidence constantly. She stated, "The strength in a limb may depend upon the confidence in which it is used."

She does a wonderful job of describing the trajectory of what she calls *nervous illness*, which I believe to be quite applicable for those with sensitized nervous systems due to medication injury or withdrawal. The trajectory she lays out begins with a sense of *indecisiveness* that leads to one being highly *suggestible*, both to outside opinions and to their own negative self-talk. This indecisive and highly suggestible person now begins to *lose confidence* in themselves, and over time, they experience what she describes as *personality disintegration*. Simply put, the individual no longer feels whole, coherent, or comfortable in their skin. This leads to *a sense of unreality*, which can often be experienced as depersonalization and derealization. It is then common for one to develop obsessions and have a mind that can get quite sticky. This *sticky* mind can lead to intrusive thoughts or looping, repetitive thoughts that can be extremely distressing. This then leads to a sense of *apathy*, followed by *depression* or *depletion*. Dr. Weekes saw depression as the natural outcome in the trajectory, as the individual feels extremely mentally fatigued and depleted. This trajectory mimics my own experience. But it was my loss of confidence that truly tipped the scales and began the rapid decline in terms of my own sense that I could or would find a way to survive.

I want to return to Dr. Weeke's comment, "The strength in a limb may depend upon the confidence in which it is used."

When I was 29 years old, I slipped while walking into a store and broke my elbow. I had to go in for emergency surgery. When I came out, the doctor informed me that my arm would most likely always hang at an angle and that with physical therapy, I could probably regain 60-65% use of it again. I was shocked and devastated. It was my right arm, and I was right-handed. I couldn't write, type, drive, or play sports.

I dove into my physical therapy. I returned to work and hired a friend, who was out of a job, to be my driver. I provided home hospice at the time and traveled two to three hours a day, but I was not permitted to drive for three months. I was determined that I would heal, and despite the pain, I knew I had to work that arm in order to have the best chance of healing. Six months later, the orthopedic surgeon was shocked that I had regained 90% use and strength in my arm and elbow. He also said, "You will find that your elbow and your arm are now stronger than ever."

This was an elbow. That is far different than our brain and central nervous system, but the same logic still applies. Somehow, we have to find that happy medium, that sweet spot, where we are pushing ourselves just enough to manifest healing, but not so hard that we create a setback or further injury. There is a great deal of trial and error in this process. In fact, since there is no real consensus in the literature about what has happened to us, our healing is virtually all trial and error. This can be cumbersome and frustrating.

How much exercise is helpful versus how much exacerbates my symptoms? What foods can I tolerate and what tends to make things worse? What shows, music, books, friends, conversations, activities can I participate in, and to what extent?

The list for our trials and errors is extensive. But to build confidence and use our brains and nervous systems in a healthy, productive manner, we must continue trying things out. Like the men on the boats with the yellow slickers, we need to throw away the starfish and sea debris as quickly as possible. Simultaneously, we need to collect the patterns of behavior as well as potentially a shift in attitude and core beliefs that will help us achieve our goal. The goal is to heal and develop healthy bio-psycho-social-spiritual scar tissue that leaves us stronger and more resilient than before.

One of my favorite books is *DARE* by Barry McDonagh. *DARE* stands for the four-part process Barry describes in his book: Defuse, Allow/Accept, Run towards, and Engage. While *DARE* was not written specifically for those grappling with a medication injury, I found the approach quite helpful. It is very similar to the works by Dr. Claire Weekes, and it seeks to encourage folks to defuse their fear by naming it: *this is just an uncomfortable sensation, just a thought, just a feeling, so what, who cares?* *DARE* then asks that you stop fighting your anxiety, fear, and difficult situation and accept and allow it to be there. Then, instead of running away from, withdrawing, or avoiding, you step into and towards your fear. If you fear leaving your home, you practice taking baby steps out the door. These small steps help you engage in your life and not let your anxiety or symptoms rule you. I have found periods of great success by employing the wisdom of Dr. Claire Weekes, *DARE* coaches Michelle Cavanaugh and Aida Beco, my beloved therapist, Sandra, and a few others, such as Paige Pradko, Sally Winston, Martin Seif, Chris Paige, Jennifer Leigh, David Powers, Michael Priebe, Geraldine Burns, and DE Foster, to name a few. By taking daily steps outside of my comfort zone and realizing I was uncomfortable, but not in any real, immediate danger, I slowly started to engage in my life a bit more freely. This is a daily practice, and there are moments when the symptoms are just too severe. But each time I try, I build back a bit of that lost confidence and move a tad further along in my healing process.

Chapter Fifteen

SCIENCE THE SHIT OUT OF IT

"I learned a long time ago the wisest thing I can do is be on my own side, be an advocate for myself and others like me."

- Maya Angelou

There is a great line from the movie *The Martian*, starring Matt Damon. On one of my low days, I stumbled upon this movie. I found deep inspiration from it. There is one line that compelled me to literally sit up and say, "Yes!" It came at a time in the movie where Matt Damon's character, having been stranded on Mars, is about to run out of food and water. He looks defeated and scared, but suddenly, it's as if he remembers who he is—a scientist, a fearless innovator who has gone into space. He says to himself, "Okay, I am going to science the shit out of this!"

In that moment, I realized that while there was more support and information for those suffering from medication injury and/or benzodiazepine withdrawal syndrome than ever before, I was still kind of out there in no-man's land. No one would show up, roll up their sleeves, and say, "Jennifer, you are too special to let wither away. We will figure this out, come hell or high water."

Yes, I had *many* people who cared and were concerned. Still, at that moment, I realized I needed to be like Matt Damon's character in *The Martian*. And, recalling another favorite movie quote, I needed to, "Get busy living or get busy dying" (said by Morgan Freeman's character Red from *The Shawshank Redemption*).

So I got busy *sciencing the shit* out of myself. While I needed to summon the troops—my support systems—I first needed to acknowledge I was the captain of those troops, this was my mission, and it was up to me.

So, again, I can't offer medical advice, but here are some things I learned as I scienced the shit out of myself:

1. Be your own advocate; ask the questions; do the research.

In my research about struggling to come off the alprazolam, I stumbled upon a detail that made my blood run cold. Professor Ashton, years prior, cautioned using fluoroquinolones while either taking or withdrawing from benzos. As you can imagine, this point grabbed my interest.

While I had not been on a benzo back in 2016 when I was given the antibiotic, I had used a small dose just two weeks prior to getting *floxed*. For years, if I had a long flight, I used a tiny dose of Xanax to help with flight anxiety and motion sickness. While the benzo should have been long out of my system, it was interesting to read an article written by Brad Verret about the risks of interaction between that class of antibiotics and benzodiazepines. He speculated that this particular class of antibiotic could potentially strip the GABA-A receptor site, thus throwing patients into acute benzo withdrawal. My symptoms of being *floxed* were nearly identical to that of someone going through acute benzo withdrawal. Yet, not one of the seven specialists in 2016, nor any of the number of doctors I saw in 2020, made or saw a possible connection.

I also learned that taking NSAIDs (Motrin, Advil, etc.) while taking a fluoroquinolone could lead to adverse reactions. Remember my hairdresser who took an NSAID for a headache and woke up in a world of hurt?

Neither the doctor at the urgent care nor the pharmacist asked me if I was taking a benzo or using an NSAID when I was prescribed the antibiotic. While I wasn't taking the former, I had taken large doses of the latter to combat a fever both the day I started my antibiotic and for a few days following discontinuation of the antibiotic.

Did taking the small dose of Xanax eight days before the antibiotics leave me more vulnerable to having an adverse reaction? Had I been given informed consent about the interactions with benzodiazepines or NSAIDs, I would have opted out of taking the antibiotic. While I am not advocating to turn to Dr. Google, as that alone can lead you down endless rabbit holes, I am advocating for slowing down, doing some research, and asking all the questions you need in order to provide fully informed consent.

Even then, it still may not save you from being a *three-to-five percenter*. Doctors aren't gods, and there are always outliers. But after listening to and reading thousands of personal accounts of these *three-to-five percenter*s, the supposed outliers, I have realized that I need to do my very best to make sure I know what I am putting in my body.

We have to be our own advocates and have someone we trust to act as one if we cannot. Until I ran into the gem of an ENT, each specialist I saw told me, "I have heard of spontaneous tendon ruptures and things like that, but nothing like you are suggesting." First of all, not *suggesting*, EXPERIENCING! Second, had my doctor or pharmacist said, "Okay, I can write you a script for something, but you need to know that there is a Black Box warning about spontaneous tendon rupture," I would have taken my sore throat and headache home or asked for something else. Not to mention, by the time I ingested those three toxic pills in September of 2016, the FDA Advisory Committee had deemed it too risky a medication for the very thing it was prescribed. There were even two Black Box warnings indicating the potential to develop the very symptoms I experienced.

In March of 2020, a few months following the surgery that kicked off the second episode, I was off work. I had just shut down my practice due to my extreme reaction to starting a rapid taper of alprazolam. I was trying to make myself walk. At the time, I was having a few good hours where I felt I could leave the house. While I walked around the neighborhood, feeling intermittently terrified that I might dissociate and get lost, I found myself hitting one of those *angry* moments. I went home and decided to contact 12 pharmacies in the surrounding area. I asked to speak to the pharmacist and said that I had a sinus infection, had gone to an urgent care center, and was given a prescription for levofloxacin, the generic form of Levaquin. I told them I didn't know much about the medication and was leery of taking things. I asked if they thought it was appropriate for a sinus infection and what I need to know about contraindications with any over-the-counter medications. ONE. ONE. ONE of the 12 pharmacists told me, "Absolutely not—this is like taking a fire extinguisher to put out a candle." They told me about the tendon ruptures—two others mentioned this too but said it was incredibly rare. He went on to ask me if I was on any other meds, specifically a benzodiazepine. You can imagine who my new pharmacist is now, right? But I was dumbstruck. Granted, this is not a gold-standard, empirically-based experiment by any means. However, only one in 12 pumped the brakes, gave me accurate information, and was uncomfortable filling the script.

We cannot assume that we will be provided with the information to make an informed decision. It is up to us to ask, ask again, and research.

I am not insinuating that doctors are purposefully withholding information to keep us from having informed consent. I don't think any doctor, whether they were able to help me or not, was coming from a place of malice. However, having many doctor friends, I am acutely aware of how challenging it is to practice medicine these days. The pressure to see a certain number of patients, as well as the litigiousness of our society, creates the expectation for them to be gods and not make any mistakes. Being expected by your medical group or hospital to see 40-60 patients per day makes it nearly impossible to slow down and thoroughly review with each patient the possible adverse effects and Black Box warnings on each medication being prescribed. In fact, many of the physicians I saw in my clinical practice were struggling to "keep up" in their lives given the near super-human demands placed on them by the institutions that employed them. In addition, many adverse reactions occur in the minority of individuals taking a particular medication. I am sure many more people are helped by fluoroquinolones, nerve medications, and benzodiazepines than harmed by them.

However, this brings me to a larger question I have for the medical community. How many narratives and anecdotal stories have to rack up for it to become empirically-based evidence? Many of the specialists I consulted said *there is just anecdotal evidence,* meaning there were just people's stories. But when you look at these groups and see patterns of debilitating symptoms affecting hundreds of thousands of people, then at what point are there enough stories to become worthy of being considered and counted as *science*?

2. Ask your doctor about genetic testing.

Some great tools available offer a blueprint to help our doctors and us identify the best medications for us. There are many, but I used the Genomind testing to obtain information about psychotropic medications that I may have a harder time metabolizing or cause an adverse response. Through this testing, I learned Valium, often used as a substitute for Xanax in a taper, was not a good fit for me. This is not to say that my genetic profile would have told me how I would have reacted to a fluoroquinolone, but it offers a great deal of information about how we metabolize medications, which can help your team identify the best path forward, specific to your body.

If you have been injured by a medication, it is imperative to find a team that both believes you and is willing to work with you. For example, the psychiatrist in 2020 recognized I was very ill from the combination of surgery, discontinuing gabapentin cold turkey, and my benzodiazepine rapid taper. She slowed me down to build my body back up via nutrition and supplements before we resumed a slow and steady benzo-taper. She was open to hearing the input and advice my internist was offering. I would often send emails to both to keep them updated and on the same page. I know I got lucky. I know how hard it is to find a doctor, let alone a team, that can invest the amount of time needed to get to the bottom of our challenging situation. Join online groups and ask if there are doctors in your city or area that someone else found helpful. If I hadn't kept pushing and looking, I wouldn't have found my team. It is very challenging while sick to have to push so hard and even say *no thank you* to well-meaning clinicians when they advise us to do things that we feel are not in our best interest.

CHAPTER SIXTEEN

MEDITATION AND MINDFULNESS PRACTICE

"Mindfulness is a way of befriending ourselves and our experience."

- Jon Kabat Zinn

Let me start by saying loud and clear that I truly stink at meditating. I have been trying to slay this elusive dragon for years, but it just won't surrender to me. This is what I have learned about meditation. It is not a dragon to slay; it is not the elusive Loch Ness monster that I will never find. That has been my problem. It isn't a destination. Before you sock me over the head with, "Jen, don't you dare offer the platitude of 'it's the journey that counts,'" just know that, in my case, this is a truth. It is a practice. There's that word again! I have been practicing for years, and I still suck. It kind of reminds me of when I was a kid and took guitar lessons. One day, I remember my guitar teacher telling my mom, "She's just not good." That probably didn't happen quite that way, but that is what my eight-year-old brain heard and remembered. I would practice, albeit intermittently and never with determination. Then, every Tuesday, I would go to my lesson, and I would suck ass as much as I had the week before. If I use that childhood experience as a lesson, two things have been problematic with my practice of meditation. It is something I only have done intermittently and without much determination. More importantly, I would only tend to implement it when I didn't feel well. If I were having a good day, the last thing I would think about was meditating. But on a bad day, I would meditate for hours. I'd do a guided body scan, listen to several guided anxiety meditations, listen to some gratitude meditations, and wonder, *Why am I not feeling better???*

First, we need to remember meditation is a practice that we do with regularity. It is not a quick fix. In fact, for some people, it isn't a fix at all. Many of my clients have shared that meditation was just not a tool that they felt they could implement for various reasons.

Let's back up a moment to clarify that mindfulness and meditation are not the same thing. The practice of meditation is a mindfulness exercise, but not all mindfulness is meditation as we know it. I like to describe mindfulness as an umbrella term that is filled with hundreds of exercises and practices that are designed to bring our attention to the present moment. We can eat mindfully, walk mindfully, pet our animals mindfully, speak to our friends mindfully, and even speak to ourselves mindfully.

For example, the process that Dr. Claire Weekes described to help with anxiety and panic was a mindfulness practice. Notice that you are in an anxious pattern, remind yourself that these are just thoughts, feelings, and experiences, work to float alongside them as you accept and allow them to be there, and let some time pass as you resume with your life. This is mindfulness. Not, *If only this feeling would leave,* or *Oh no! I was doing so well. How could I be feeling like this again!?*

Another mindfulness practice is breathwork. I stumbled upon the work of Max Strom during my second episode, and I bought his online program to teach myself a way to breathe through my challenges. I had gone 50 years breathing. But I never really learned how to breathe properly and certainly never how to breathe diaphragmatically to help aid my emotional distress. I loved his work and found the breathwork to be incredibly helpful.

For others, it's yoga, gardening, going for a walk, being out in nature, stopping to smell or taste or feel or listen. But remember the important point: **we get good at what we practice.** During my first and second episodes, I practiced self-pity a lot, and guess what? I got really good at it. On my bad days, I practiced panic. Guess what I got good at?

While I still suck at meditating, I found a few helpful things. I listen to and do Jon Kabat Zinn's guided body scan often. His voice is soothing, and he asks, in the beginning, to just be where we are and to not work so hard to be where we are not. We don't want to be there when we don't feel well. Here is the only real place we can be. The past and future don't exist any longer or yet. We are where we are.

For sleep meditation, I found a 45-minute recording of Tony Shaloub reading *A Short Account of the History of Mathematics.* It was incredibly rare for me to hear the end of that recording. Hearing Tony talk about fractions and various periods of time as mathematics evolved was enough to put me right out. I found that I couldn't drift off if I listened to anything I hadn't heard before or something I was interested in. Thank you, Tony and mathematics. A man I adore and a subject I abhor. You have helped me more than you know.

Another group of online videos that I found to be professional and helpful are by Paige Pradko, and are available for free on YouTube. Paige uses a method she developed called the CALM method. CALM is an acronym for 1) Calm your mind, 2) Accept your anxiety, 3) Logic, and 4) Moving on. She pulls from various evidence-based strategies, such as Cognitive Behavioral Therapy, Dialectical Behavioral Therapy, and Acceptance and Commitment Therapy. She does an excellent job teaching diaphragmatic breathing with a great square breathing tool, progressive muscle relaxation, and breathing meditation. Along with this comprehensive four-part method, Paige also has excellent information on intrusive thoughts, worry, and other helpful videos related to all aspects of anxiety. She also recently released two online programs that I have found incredibly informative and helpful. One is called "Rapid Recovery from Health Anxiety," and the other is "Free from Pure O and OCD." While not a benzo coach/therapist specifically, Paige is very open, aware, and has seen firsthand the various manifestations of anxiety, including depersonalization/derealization, obsessive thoughts, intrusive thoughts, fear, phobias, panic, hypervigilance, and health anxiety that arise in benzodiazepine withdrawal.

Another helpful resource is the website and YouTube videos of David Powers. David is a PhD candidate in psychology who went through his own challenging recovery from benzodiazepine withdrawal ten years ago. He offers great insight and practical advice through his eBook, *The Powers Manual*. The manual describes a two-part process referred to as *pushing and lulling*. Meditation, breathwork, and mindfulness activities are a few things that he incorporates in his *lulling* approach.

I've had many people well versed in the art of mindfulness gently remind me not to get caught up in trying to find *the right way* to meditate or engage in mindfulness practice. There is no one right or wrong way. Downward dog stretches, flame meditations, counting your steps, diaphragmatic breathing, fully and mindfully experiencing your mashed potatoes, or listening to Tony talk fractions on Audible... there are countless ways out there to both become present moment focused and ease our weary minds.

CHAPTER SEVENTEEN

FEAR OF BANANAS

*"Everywhere is within walking
distance if you have the time."*

- Steven Wright

I don't know if this is only for people who have been *floxed* or folks in benzo withdrawal, but wildly irrational fears abound in this process. Let me restate this. It would *appear* that the fears are irrational—some are, some aren't. When you have been injured by a prescribed medication, when you have followed the rules and still been burned, it is hard to trust. There is a trauma in realizing that even when doing everything right, your life can still be turned upside down.

With this distrust comes quite a bit of hypervigilance. Things that you took for granted now seem suspect, and everything has the potential to harm you. For example, I learned that artificial sweeteners, sugar, caffeine, soy, and dairy all seemed to make me feel worse. Supplements that I would have never second-guessed taking pre-injury—vitamin D, an iron supplement, some vitamin C, magnesium—all became potential villains in my process of healing.

I began to fear food. I had heard bone broth was good for healing the gut. I started making my own bone broth and drinking it a few times a day. Then, one day, I woke up covered in hives and with terrible headaches. Soon, I learned that bone broth, especially the way I was making it, is super high in histamines. Coming off of certain medications can destabilize your mast cells, causing histamine reactions.

I explained my hives and newfound fear of bone broth to my dear friend who was also in benzo withdrawal, and she admitted, "I know what you mean. I am afraid of bananas."

It takes *a lot* to make me laugh when I feel like I am hanging on by a thread. But when my friend admitted she feared bananas, I laughed so hard I thought I would come unglued. So, my fear of bone broth and her fear of bananas (also a potential histamine releaser) were not necessarily irrational. They were founded in the trauma of having had a bad reaction. But it became essential to try to reign in my fears a bit. I couldn't be afraid to try a different vegetable or fruit for fear that it would set off my symptoms.

What I had to learn the *hard way* was too much of anything can be bad.

CHAPTER EIGHTEEN

HOW DO I EAT? HOW DO I MOVE? HOW DO I REST?

"Happiness is not a matter of intensity but of balance and order and rhythm and harmony."

- Thomas Merton

This is a big one. Learning how to eat, hydrate, move, and rest to heal myself has been a huge learning curve. However, it has forever changed me in my professional work. I now listen intently and with deep clinical curiosity when someone discusses how they eat, drink, sleep, and move. These factors are imperative in one's quality of life and healing process.

I won't launch into a full discussion of the role that epigenetics play in the manner in which we find ourselves in a state of health or illness, but do yourself a favor and look into this booming field of study. Epigenetics looks at the way in which our environment (our external environment, our behaviors, and our internal belief systems) interplays with our genetic make-up by literally turning "on" and "off" our genes. So the way we eat, hydrate, sleep, move, the quality of our relationships, and the manner in which we navigate stress are all epigenetic factors that interact with how our genetic coding manages both the creation of and maintenance of illness and how we heal.

I changed aspects of my diet and lifestyle after my first episode with the antibiotic. However, once it seemed behind me for the most part, I did NOT want to be reminded. I went through the next few years somewhat afraid of medications but pretty much avoiding the reality of how bad it had been. I convinced myself that I was just fine. I went back to my regular diet (not great, but not horrible), began to drink socially again, and I could have exercised more. Whenever I had a problem falling asleep, I was afraid; those nights spent watching the minutes tick by for a year and a half were excruciating. But I was sleeping again by the 18th month after the incident, so I never gave that much mind. The only thing I did not return to after the 2016 episode was caffeine.

In episode two, it was clear that healing would require some dramatic changes. Over six weeks, I cut off all processed foods, sugar (except from fruit), gluten, dairy, soy, and alcohol. (I don't recommend someone making these dramatic changes so quickly.) My doctor had me start on some supplements; however, using supplements while coming off benzodiazepines is highly controversial, and many feel much worse on them. At the beginning of my taper, the supplements worked well. However, I learned the hard way that they can sneak up on you and ruin even the best of plans. A few months prior to writing this book, I had to hold my benzo-taper for several months as I tapered off various supplements that were suddenly getting in the way of my recovery.

I began to drink nothing other than water and fresh ginger tea (just raw, organic ginger steeped in hot water), and LOTS of it.

I took a probiotic to try to keep my gut health in check, took garlic pills to act as a natural antibiotic, and a product called d-mannose to help keep away urinary tract infections (UTI), as I was entering perimenopause, and UTIs can often be more common.

My sleep was helped by an anti-depressant I was put on well before I really knew much about benzodiazepine recovery. While it did help with sleep, looking back, I would have opted not to put another medication in my system. It will be one more thing I'll eventually have to deal with. Depression and sleep issues are a common part of benzodiazepine withdrawal and are manageable, but please slow down to consider if adding more medications to your experience is warranted, justified, and necessary.

Exercise has also been key to my recovery. This can be very hard to do when you are feeling terrible. It can also be impossible to do if your medication injury has left you with ruptured tendons, muscle or bone pain, or a myriad of other complicating factors. If you can move, do it. Not only will the movement help as a natural detox for your body, but it will provide a natural release of endorphins and hormones to help with mood and sleep too. I have met many along the way for whom *moving* meant walking to their mailbox and back. If that is all you can do, do it. For others, the medication injury set them on a health and exercise journey they would never have attempted otherwise. Last night, I spoke to a guy who, amid his acute withdrawal, walked ten miles a day to help with his restlessness and agitation. A few weeks ago, I spoke to someone else who was in withdrawal, agoraphobic, and in terrible pain but would still make sure she walked 20 laps around the inside of her home every day. Even on my worst days, I feel better even if I can make a few house laps or march in place. We do what we can.

When the antibiotic first injured me, once I got over my irrational fear of drowning, I found that being outside in the open air was incredibly helpful for my overall mood and sense of self. There is something healing about getting out from beyond your four walls. Do what you can. For many of us, our brains will tell us, *What's the point?* or *I can't go for a walk, I can barely make myself something to eat.* We get good at what we practice. Period. What I found was that if I could just challenge myself to do a little something more each day, just tiptoe out of my comfort zone, I could usually succeed. These can be the simplest things. One day, it was washing my bedsheets. Later, it was meeting a family member or friend for dinner. And it is not always a linear thing; right now, it's back to just washing the bedsheets. Even so, these small successes help our sense of self and can build on each other to form the new skin that we will find ourselves in as we heal.

CHAPTER NINETEEN

CHEMICAL ANXIETY, DEPRESSION, DP/DR, AND INTRUSIVE THOUGHTS

*"But what we call our despair is often
only the painful eagerness of unfed hope."*

- George Eliot

E ven the title of this chapter yields a visceral shudder in me as I type. This will be a bit of a longer chapter as there is, unfortunately, much for me to say about my experience with these symptoms. I never thought or even heard of the concept of chemical anxiety or depression prior to these medication injuries. It is impossible for me to describe how this feels. In fact, it makes me kind of sick to my stomach just thinking about trying to explain it. Chemical anxiety and depression are different beasts than anything I had ever experienced before. I had times in my life when I struggled with a bit of depression or anxiety. But what I felt after the antibiotic fiasco, and what I have continued to face throughout my benzo-taper, is like comparing hurricanes to light summer rains.

It's important to note, however, that I am not minimizing those experiencing anxiety not brought on by the discontinuation of a medication or a benzodiazepine. I have met many folks, especially in my DARE community, who describe quite similar experiences and symptoms—both physical and mental—to what I am going through in my withdrawal. It was precisely that reason that led me to believe that the DARE program might have some tools to benefit me in my recovery, and I have found that to be the case.

This is probably an important place to pause and elaborate a bit. Even though I was not placed on a benzodiazepine for anxiety, in my discontinuation of the medication, I have experienced nearly every manifestation of anxiety as well as symptoms that would earn me a DSM-5 diagnosis of many other psychiatric conditions. This point becomes very important on many fronts. But for the purposes of this chapter, I have found it very important to really research great resources related to anxiety and depression, as well as skilled-based approaches, such as DBT, forms of CBT, and ACT, to create for myself a tool-kit to navigate this experience and all of its "pop up, kick me in gut" array of sensations, thoughts, and feelings.

I refer to my anxiety and depression as "chemical" only because they were induced by a medication discontinuation and were not clinically present before that process. Some would argue that the level of anxiety, depression, and symptoms we experience in withdrawal are much more intense than those that grapple with these issues who are not in an active withdrawal process. I would say it really doesn't matter. I have met many folks who are bed bound, housebound, agoraphobic, monophobic, have unrelenting panic, painful body sensations, and are tormented by intrusive thoughts that were not in the middle of a complicated, hellish medication withdrawal. So, since so little is written or available to and for those of us in withdrawal, I went to the places and the people that were helping those souls grappling with similar symptoms while not in withdrawal and began to build my toolkit. It didn't matter if my sensitization and anxiety was med induced, I was still in pain. And comparing pain is like comparing love. It is highly subjective. What is the greatest love? The love you feel. What is the greatest pain? The pain you feel. So, while I recognize I am in the middle of a giant neurochemical shit storm in my central nervous system, I have also found great relief and support in looking at other more established areas of study to gain some tools. While there are a handful of coaches who have been through benzo withdrawal, and I have found talking to each of them incredibly helpful, there is also a wealth of information and knowledge for helping non med-injured folks learn how to navigate extreme anxiety and all of its mental and physical manifestations. All of these resources I found helpful are discussed throughout the book as well as in the resource list at the back.

A sense of sheer terror often accompanied my chemical anxiety. And I'm not just talking about a fear of bananas and bone broth, I'm referring to a blood-curdling sense of terror that is unexplainable. Sometimes, it may be the sensation that something was inside of me, trying to come out through my stomach and up through my throat. It was all-consuming. Sometimes, it was an internal shiver and a sense that I could not calm myself no matter what I did. Mentally, it often took the form of both monophobia and agoraphobia. Monophobia is the fear of being alone. I didn't want someone to come and entertain me. I just needed to know another adult was in the next room or down the hall. I went through a particularly rough stretch and actually hired someone to be with me during the day for a while. Again, not to tend to me, but it was comforting to know someone was there. I also had bouts of agoraphobia when I feared going out in public—running to the grocery store, taking a walk, and even visiting with family. However, because this entire second episode has coincided with COVID, my desire to have groceries delivered, hesitancy to go out to dinner, and desire to remain at home has not stood out as odd.

I have talked to many people in withdrawal who also struggled with monophobia and agoraphobia. What nearly everyone describes is that it eventually dissipates, and they can resume their normal level of social functioning. More than once, I have been told, "If it came in with withdrawal, it will leave with withdrawal." Dr. Claire Weekes has an interesting take on agoraphobia. She does not feel it is an actual phobia (irrational fear of something specific), as it is not the actual fear of being outside of the home. Instead, it is the fear that one will experience panic or symptoms as they are out of the home and feel out of control, ashamed, or embarrassed. Her simple (but not easy) approach of facing the fear/panic, floating, and letting time pass applies to agoraphobia, as it does to other forms of anxiety.

For me, chemical depression took the form of literal heavy, black clouds that would swoop in out of nowhere and take me down. I could be doing just fine, just watching a movie or doing some work, and suddenly it was upon me. A sense of dread. A fatigue both mental and physical. A sense of hopelessness. When these clouds would wash over me, I was terrified. I would reach out to my support and ask them, "Am I clinically depressed?" And they would remind me that just the day before, I had been out at a baseball game, watching my nephew and laughing. Or that even earlier that same day, I had been on the phone and felt fine. That is how quickly and how consuming these waves of chemical anxiety and depression can be.

Often, my chemical depression would lead to various obsessions, a series of scary *What ifs?* I love Dr. Weekes' clear and simple understanding of these obsessive worries. She simply says they are nothing more than *strange thoughts in a tired mind*. I cannot tell you the thousands of times I have repeated those words when I find myself overcome with obsessional worry or fear.

DP/DR. Ugh. Here is a true beast. Depersonalization (DP) and derealization (DR) exist on a spectrum, just like anxiety and depression. At times they can be uneasy background noise; other times, they border on a psychotic level of functioning. Depersonalization is the sense that you are not real. Derealization is the sense that other things are not real. For me, they often go hand in hand. They could swoop in out of nowhere. I could be talking to a friend or my mom and suddenly feel out of my body, unsure if it were really me talking, a terrifying level of self-fragmentation.

Strangely, it seemed to happen the most when I would be watching a movie. One night, I was in a good space, watching a documentary on the college admissions scandal. Halfway through, a dark, menacing, fragmenting force came over me. I spent a half-hour feeling there, but not there, terrified but afraid to move, unsure if it was really me watching the movie, and feeling that I might lose my mind. I immediately reached out to a friend who had been through benzo withdrawal years before, and she said, "What is the background music like?" I hadn't even noticed the background music. She said, "Is it melancholic or intense?" I went back to the movie, listened, and sure enough, there was dark, intense music underlying the content of the documentary. She said, "Gets me every time. I get DP/DR'd out of my mind with some documentaries, shows, and even commercials."

I have since realized that my chemical terror and DP/DR can certainly intensify with certain sounds or music. Those of us facing central nervous system injuries are incredibly sensitive, and things that would never have bothered us in the least in our prior lives can suddenly be overwhelming, disorienting, and terrifying.

Shaun O'Connor has a wonderful manual and videos for purchase at www.dpmanual.com. Shaun suffered from DP and anxiety. He spent years researching to create a straightforward, compassionate, no-nonsense approach to managing this particular distressing manifestation of anxiety. I listened to his audiobook repeatedly and would return to particular chapters in moments when I began to feel overwhelmed by my own DP.

Not only does he have a very calming voice, his system just makes sense.

Barry McDonagh's DARE team also has some great resources and a video on YouTube that I found incredibly helpful. I also found the YouTube videos by Jordan Hardgrave to be very articulate and informative as well. Drew Linsalata has a great podcast and has also written a few books that describe his journey with intense anxiety and how he practiced and learned to navigate and quell his struggle. Just as Dr. Weekes had used her own experience of anxiety to write her groundbreaking books, it is reassuring to know that Shaun, Jordan, Drew, and Barry, along with his DARE team, have also walked this scary and confusing ground ahead of us. They have come out the other side and are able to provide us with hard-won knowledge and guidance.

The strangest and one of the hardest symptoms for me are intrusive thoughts. They started with that original thought that I would drown myself in the swimming pool after being *floxed* in 2016. Intrusive thoughts are simply that: intrusive, unwanted, and often dystonic. By dystonic, I mean these thoughts are not in line with your healthy thinking, values, or beliefs about yourself. Some fear losing their mind, committing suicide, or hurting someone else. Some describe disgusting or vile sexual or violent thoughts that leave them wondering if they are morally flawed. Some have thoughts about stealing or going to jail. For others, the thoughts can be simply strange but benign, like, *Is my dog real?* Intrusive thoughts happen to everyone—not just us injured folk. *What if I stepped off this ledge?* or *What if I pushed that person off that ledge?* are common examples. But for those of us with injured or sensitive nervous systems, these thoughts can send us into a whole cascade of hurt.

In the book *Overcoming Unwanted Intrusive Thoughts,* Dr. Sally Winston and Dr. Martin Seif describe a common experience felt as a *whoosh* that accompanies an intrusive thought. For me, I would feel this *whoosh* both mentally and physically. I would have the thought, my body would physically react with a fear response (like a flush), and I would feel fear followed by a more intense physical response, followed by more fear, until it felt incapacitating.

For many people, they have an intrusive thought, have a mild physical or emotional reaction to it, realize, *Damn, that was strange,* and resume their daily life, knowing they would not act on it. It was simply a thought. For those of us with CNS injuries, we don't recover nearly as fast as the average person. Due to our tired minds and injured brains (amygdala/frontal cortex, etc.), we are more susceptible to what Seif and Winston refer to as *sticky mind.* As thoughts enter our minds that are not in line with our values or how we see ourselves, we experience a dramatic *whoosh.* Once the *whoosh* sets in mentally and physically, our bell is now rung. We are in mental and physical distress, which creates fear, which exacerbates the mental and physical reaction, which reinforces the fear, and round and round we go.

Much like Dr. Claire Weekes' model of fear-adrenaline-fear-adrenaline that keeps the fear/anxiety/obsession alive, Seif and Winston describe a similar process. Those with a sticky mind have an unwanted thought, which leads to the *whoosh*, which is then often responded to with a sense of fear, disgust, shame, or guilt leading to an urgent attempt to suppress the thought or rationalize it away. This suppression, avoidance, or search for reassurance has a paradoxical effect and leads to the thought becoming more stuck and looping. The more the thought is stuck and looping, the more likely we become convinced that the thought must have relevance and deeper meaning. And round and round we go, often feeling like we are losing our minds or falling into a deep sense of despair.

I have dug a deeper hole for myself in my own struggle with intrusive thoughts by becoming a reassurance junkie. I would talk with friends, family, or my therapist to be reassured that these thoughts were not reflective of me or some unresolved issue in my life. Seif and Winston view seeking reassurance as counterproductive because in doing so, you are acting as if the thought has relevance or meaning. This simply tells the brain to continue sounding the alarm. They propose a counter-intuitive stance; rather than exerting *more* effort to replace, understand, or squelch the thought, they advocate that less is more. We are to take a bird's eye view, recognize that the content is irrelevant, and leave it alone. That said, as I stated earlier, we often need good information first to then begin to employ this counter-intuitive response of, "Oh well!" or "So what?" in relation to our symptoms. This is why Claire Weekes says repeatedly in her books, "I am assuming you have been checked out by a physician and you have been told it is nerves."

Medication injury and withdrawal can mimic many, many ailments. So, of course, you want to be sure you aren't ignoring a heart problem, a thyroid issue, or a back injury that might have presented regardless of your current withdrawal situation. That said, once we get that confirmation, we have to stay off Dr. Google and practice not putting our uncomfortable symptoms under a microscope or meeting them a hundred times a day with "if only" or "what if."

Seif and Winston offer a powerful system to help us manage our intrusive thoughts. They utilize the phrase, "Robert Just Ate Fries, Tacos, and Pies" as a way of remembering the model. We *recognize* that we are having an intrusive thought. We label them as *just* thoughts (not going to hurt us and are not facts). We don't seek to avoid or squelch them but instead *accept and allow* them in. They are here and nothing to be frightened about. We allow ourselves to *float freely* alongside them, while letting *time pass,* and ultimately *proceed* with our daily tasks.

I have tried this, and it works. Again, it's a practice. Our minds realize that we aren't going to fight the thoughts. They grasp that we won't be interrupted by the thoughts for long and that we actually have a system to manage them. As a result, they eventually do calm down.

Dr. Jennifer Leigh, a benzo coach who also writes a blog, has been very transparent about intrusive thoughts being one of the roughest symptoms in her recovery. I had several conversations with her and found her approach to be gentle, effective, and normalizing.

One thing that has been incredibly helpful to me in both understanding and accepting all of the distressing symptoms I mention above has been to really study our biology and our neurochemistry. This has allowed me to gain some insight into the actual mechanics of our stress response system. What is happening in the Limbic system, what is going on in the interplay of our amygdala and our hypothalamus and our HPA axis (hypothalamus-pituitary-adrenals)? As I spent hours studying and learning, I realized that most of my terrible thoughts, sensations, and feelings were a result of my stress response system trying to protect me, but things had gone haywire due to an injured/overtaxed and raw nervous system. I also realized that my *Oh no, I hate how I feel* reaction was pressing my stress response system to continue to misfire stress hormones and was potentially keeping many of my symptoms activated. As I have noted time and again, I am not an MD, not a neuroscientist, and not a biochemist. However, if you are interested in learning more about my armchair ponderings and revelations about this, you can look at a few videos on my YouTube channel at jenniferswanphd, where I discuss our stress response system (the videos are "Lions and Tigers and Bears," "Anxiety in Benzo Withdrawal," "What's Happening to Us," and "What the Hell is Happening"). I also have a couple videos specific to intrusive thoughts. Once we start understanding some degree of why we are feeling what we are feeling, we have to move into the practice of "smart efforts" toward not making things worse.

There are two strategies that I recently started to incorporate and have found helpful. The first is simply what I called, "Yep, got the email, thanks!" When I am struggling with very challenging and highly distressing physical sensations, rapid fire intrusive thoughts, depression, or any host of symptoms, I make myself pause and imagine them as a fire alarm going off. Now, if I were in my apartment and the fire alarm sounded, I would immediately mobilize, grab my dogs, my wallet, and my keys, and exit the complex and get to safety.

But for many of us injured by medications or in a complicated withdrawal, our fire alarms keep sounding and the thoughts, feelings, or sensations can be relentless. I now imagine and say to myself (sometimes 50 times a day!), *Jen, remember you got that email that they were testing the fire alarms in the apartment complex today? Yes, it's highly uncomfortable, it's annoying, and agitating, but there is no fire. You are not in any danger.* That is what is happening for many of us—our highly sensitized nervous systems and our misfiring stress response system are keeping us in a high state of anxiety. **The antidote to all anxiety is irrelevance.** So, I spend a lot of time thinking to myself, *Yep, we knew it was going to feel like this.* And instead of hating it and pushing it away, I work to accept it and allow it to be there. We can't FORCE the sensations to cease, but we can accept that they are there and not add fear to fear.

The second strategy I have used has been a meditation I recorded on my phone and play back to myself daily. My own voice talking to me is basically reinforcing that I am my own comfort. I am my own safe person. In this meditation, I do a sort of body scan where I begin by saying, "I accept my body and mind exactly as they are in this moment." I then do a full body scan in which I imagine a healing force entering from the soles of my feet and moving upwards through each body part, and each vital organ. I imagine this healing force healing my GABA-A receptors and working to pull all of my neurotransmitters and hormones into homeostasis. I imagine it moving through my limbic system and calming down and regulating my stress response system. I end this meditation by saying, "I am healed. It is so." While this is my own meditation, it is certainly not unique. There are many folks that talk about healing meditations, some using colors or objects or past or future images, or calling up an image of what you want to be true, such as eating dinner with your family in a restaurant or taking a trip. This is just the one that seems to be working for me. What we feed our minds matters. The mind-body connection is undeniable and doing what we can to feed our 40 trillion cells the message that we know they carry the inherent capacity to regenerate, heal, and transform can be a powerful message.

The problem with these strategies, as all things, is that they aren't a one and done sort of approach. Again, we get good at what we practice. It may take me doing this twice a day for months or a year before I feel any real healing take place. But I do believe it will work. And perhaps it is that last point that is the most powerful. I BELIEVE IT WILL WORK! Remember, it is the idea that I will see it when I believe it, not the other way around that becomes critical. I understand it can be so hard to believe when you have been suffering or struggling for months or years. I really do. But I'm banking on the equation that time plus effort equals healing. I'll keep you updated in my blog on my website and in my videos regarding how the practice of this meditation is helping or not helping me along in my healing journey.

It is important to note that while I have found many things useful, there are many days and times where the chemical onslaught and impact of the injury itself have gotten in the way of my being able to even find my tool kit, let alone be able to reach inside and grab a tool to utilize. Over time, however, I have come to find one approach that is like the "golden hammer" in my tool kit, and that is ACCEPTANCE/ALLOWANCE. Even if I can't get out of bed because the neuropathy is too great, can't think straight as my thoughts rapid fire, or can't eat because my stomach is pained and tight, I always try to remember to reach for my "golden hammer" and employ Amor Fati and my own withdrawal version of the Serenity Prayer.

My biggest obstacle isn't the sensations, the thoughts, or the feelings. I can't do anything about those. It is my FIGHT AGAINST the sensations, thoughts, or feelings. It is the story I am telling myself about it–*Oh no, I'll never get better* or *Oh no, that thought is back* or *Oh no, I will always be depressed* or *What if I never heal?* or *What if this feeling of unreality never leaves?* or *What if my POTS or my vertigo leave me bedbound forever?*

I can't do much about the movie that is playing in my mind and body, but I can remember that I am the observer of the movie. No matter how much it feels like I am starring in it, as well as being the stunt double who is getting the shit kicked out of her, I have found working to de-identify with what I am feeling, thinking, and experiencing has made a huge difference.

We are not the pain, the fear, the terror, the depression, the sensitization. Finding just that sliver of space... and believe me, I know how hard it can be to do that when you feel you are being devoured, but finding that sliver of space offers us that potential for a bit of that freedom that Frankl made reference to in his quote. The freedom to choose. Choose the narrative we tell ourselves about our experience, our fate. Choose where we place our attention. Our limbic system is watching and waiting to see whether we will react or respond. Will we fuel it further or will we choose a different way?

I did not cause this injury and it is not my fault. But withdrawal and its army made up of hundreds of bullying and brutish cousins have shown up at my doorstep. I didn't invite them, and I don't know how long they are going to stick around. I can't control them as they jump on my furniture, throw food on my floor, and play catch with my most prized possessions. If I spend my energy trying to control them, I will lose everything. If I leave and try to avoid them and abandon my house, they have won. I don't know about you guys, but I am a bit pissed and have no desire to let this bullshit evict me from my home–my body, my mind. But we have to be discerning, careful, and thoughtful about what we do with our conviction to not let withdrawal and its asshole cousins win. So, what is the best approach to get a herd of bullies to back off? Indifference. *Oh well, keep taunting me, who cares?* I won't run, I won't hide, and I won't turn and throw a punch (there's a hundred of them and I'll get pummeled). I choose what Viktor Frankl chose. I choose what James Stockdale chose. I choose what Jennifer Leigh, Baylissa, Chris Paige, David Powers, Michael Priebe, Nicole Lamberson, Christy Huff, D E Foster, Geraldine Burns, and so many others before us chose. They did what they had to do to remain vertical and breathing despite horrendous symptoms. They found the tools and resources to allow them to do so, and then they let time pass. How we encounter and engage the conflict that the withdrawal bully and his cronies are attempting to wage is critical. They may win a few battles, but we will win the war.

CHAPTER TWENTY

FEAR

"You become what you give your attention to."

- Epictetus

Although I just spoke about chemical terror, I feel that fear deserves its own chapter. For me, chemical terrors were the bolts of lightning. Fear, however, is the dark, scary, and ominous sky ridden with storm clouds. While intrusive thoughts were my worst symptom, fear was and continues to be my most pervasive.

Think of it as a sort of soup, an eerie, creepy broth that I swim around in all day, every day. At the beginning of my withdrawal journey, it would come and go. However, at some point in the last nine months, it rolled in one day and never left. I often describe myself feeling like a scared kid, no clothes, no shoes, lost and alone.

I have come to understand that this constant state of fear is simply my limbic system in a frantic state, sending up so many flares of danger in such rapid succession as to create a panoramic and constant field of danger. Like the grand finale at the end of a firework display, but the finale seems never to end. After a while, there are no more *ooooooohs* and *ahhhhhhs* from the crowd, just some head-scratching and irritation as we wonder, *When exactly is this going to be over?*

Even if I am experiencing a reprieve from strange, unwanted thoughts or moments of primal terror, I never seem to get a total reprieve or lift from this symptom. Fear has become the back-drop to my everyday life. As I go for my daily walk, I often encounter people walking their dogs, people pushing their ba-bies in strollers, people working on their lawns or their cars. Every single sight has the potential to become a grizzly bear. I *know* intellectually I am looking at a woman walking her boxer puppy or a child riding a bike, but my mind and body feel noth-ing but fear and distress. I have to talk to myself and remind myself hundreds of times a day that I am not in any danger. I say to myself over and over, *I know I am feeling fear, but it is just my mind playing tricks on me.*

Things from my past that had not been scary or strange are now remembered through the lens of fear. I hear songs or have random, benign memories pop into my head and suddenly feel a sinister, ominous, and dark feeling surrounding them. When I think about anything in the future—from going to the grocery store, getting my hair cut, or a family vacation planned two years down the road—my mind fills with fear, dread, and a warning, *You better not do that; you better not go.*

This is where the techniques that Dr. Claire Weekes and the folks at DARE describe really became a game-changer for me. Both teach not to fight fear with fear. The trap is we feel fear and all of its accordant uncomfortable thoughts, feelings, and sensations. Then, we begin to fear that feeling. On a call with Michelle Cavanaugh, a coach from the DARE program, she offered up the simple response of, "Oh f#*king well," to each and every fear-based thought, feeling, and sensation. At first, I thought this was too simplistic, but it has proven to be extremely helpful. Again, she was telling and teaching me that the antidote to anxiety and all of its scary offspring (intrusive thoughts, general sense of unease, phobias, depersonalization and derealization, etc.) is IRRELEVANCE. *That dog looks like a grizzly bear; that grocery store looks like a grizzly bear; that man fixing his car looks like a grizzly bear; my heart is palpating as if it just saw a grizzly bear; my stomach is churning as if I just ate a grizzly bear*—Oh f#*king well!

I cannot tell you what a deviation this technique was from my lifelong personal and professional tendency to stop, explore, think things through, analyze, evaluate, and problem solve. But you cannot solve a thinking problem with more thinking, and you cannot resolve your anxious state with grit or by fighting, engaging, and constantly grappling with it. Less is more. Let it go, drop the rope, stop playing the game. I still live with fear, as my limbic system is still on high alert and quite affected by my injury, but *Oh f#*king well* has changed my whole attitude towards my highly sensitized and fear-based state.

CHAPTER TWENTY-ONE

MORNING DREAD AND ANGST

"The journey of a thousand miles begins with one step."

- Lao Tzu

Holy cow. For me and many others, mornings can be unbelievably challenging. My friend Geraldine believes it is because we detox as we sleep; as a result, the first few hours we are up, we are trying to rid ourselves of these toxins. Others suggest that our cortisol is higher in the morning, so we feel shakier and more symptomatic. In both episodes of my injury/illness and recovery, I can count on probably two hands the number of mornings I have woke feeling well.

I have found it helpful to get up and get out of my bed as soon as I open my eyes. Laying there trying to fall back to sleep often yields what I refer to as *toxic sleep,* where I am in and out but ultimately feel worse. If I don't fall back into toxic sleep, I often lay there and think about my situation, and it is never with a positive frame. I will often ruminate, worry, catastrophize, and then before I know it, I have started my day from a space of major mental deficit.

Let me take a moment to clarify for any friend, loved one, or family member reading this book. I am not talking about the very common *morning blues* that some people experience as they face a long day at work or a stressful situation. This is a completely different beast and not one I would have believed had I not experienced it myself. Many wake up in a panic; others in what feels like an agitated depression. Many describe a feeling of deep dread and fear. I began to think of my mornings as a game show that I call *The Wheel of Doom*. Whether it was paralyzing terror, an adrenaline surge that literally shook me and hurt as the hormone coursed through my body, or waking to a sense of apocalyptic dread and gloom, it is consistently the worst part of my day.

Dr. Claire Weekes wrote about the need to get up and start your day. Once those eyes open, do not marinate between the sheets. This is easier said than done. At least for me, it was almost instantaneous that my mind would go to a negative space and my thoughts would begin to spin. *Here we go again—this is like Groundhog Day—I don't want to get up only to find out in a few hours I am back in hell again.* But on the days that I did practice her advice and make myself get up, make a cup of tea, have breakfast, take the pups out, go for a 15-minute walk, it made an enormous difference.

For the folks I know who struggle mightily with insomnia due to the med injury and withdrawal process, mornings may look quite a bit different. I have one friend who could never fall asleep until at least 4:00 or 5:00 a.m. each day. However, when she would get up at 10:00 or 11:00, she often described the same issues—a propensity to lay there, ruminate, worry, and catastrophize.

So, just try to put your feet on the floor, open the blinds, and start your day. Gone for me are those *lovely lazy days* when I would wake on a Saturday and think, *Oh good, I can sleep another hour or so.* My bed, albeit my safe place often in this process, can quickly become a house of horrors if I am not careful.

CHAPTER TWENTY-TWO

SFUMATO

"If uncertainty is unacceptable to you, it turns into fear.
If it is perfectly acceptable, it turns into aliveness,
alertness, and creativity."

- Eckhart Tolle

Years ago, I was reading a book about the life of Leonardo Da Vinci. The book spoke about the concept of sfumato and described it as being the "smudging technique" that he used when he painted the Mona Lisa. The implementation of sfumato is credited for why there has been so much discussion about whether the Mona Lisa is sad or happy, peaceful or in distress, even a man or a woman. Later I heard someone use the term on a broader scale and describe sfumato as the idea of comfort with ambiguity. I don't know why exactly that term captured my attention, and most who know me are aware this is one of my favorite words. Maybe because throughout my life, I have always been more comfortable and authentic in the *gray* of life rather than in the black and white, and I have never been comfortable with polarities. I like discourse, discussion, and curiosity rather than pathological certainty, and I am a fan of *this/and* rather than *either/or.*

So, *sfumato* came home to roost for me in this process of injury and recovery. Talk about having to work to get comfortable with ambiguity and uncertainty. So, let me back up a bit. While, in theory, I am all about process and *let's see how this plays out*, what I realized very quickly was that my comfort with uncertainty did not apply to me and my health. I would have paid big bucks to have a doctor be able to say, "I know exactly what has happened to you, and I have EXACTLY the protocol to make you better." I would take that pathological certainty and celebrate!

But alas, that is not the nature of a neuro-toxic injury from a medication. I learned that the brain heals in the most non-linear ways. The only thing that is predictable about healing is how unpredictable it is. One is tasked with learning and accepting that a good hour does not guarantee that the next hour will be as good. However, this works the opposite way as well. A bad hour does not mean you will get stuck there either. This makes planning quite a problem. On a Tuesday, the invitation to meet a friend sounds manageable, but by Thursday, you are benched with symptoms and know you will need to cancel only to wake up the next day and feel that you can make it. I can't tell you the number of times I have been up and down in the course of a day. The brain is strange in that if I wasn't careful, I would believe that whatever my current state of feeling was, I thought I had always felt that way or would always feel that way moving forward.

Despite tons of evidence that I moved from up to down, from feeling good to bad, functional and non-functional, when I was down, my injured brain would tell me, *This is it, this time you are down for the count. You haven't felt good in so long, and you will never feel well again.* And when I was *up,* I would tend to forget how bad it had been. I am grateful for the latter, but the former was a killer. This is why that letter to *bad self* from *good self* that I referenced earlier becomes so important.

So, sfumato shifted from a cool concept and a favorite word to my life's mission to get comfortable with uncertainty. In the benzo world, Professor Ashton spoke about benzodiazepine withdrawal and recovery in terms of windows and waves. Windows are those moments, days, weeks of clarity while one experiences a respite from the slap of symptoms. Waves are just the opposite: waves of symptoms that can swoop in and visit for a few hours or move in, kick up their dirty feet on your coffee table, and demand full attention like an unwanted, narcissistic house guest.

Again, please don't think that *getting comfortable with uncertainty* regarding our health or wellbeing is a destination or a state that we achieve. At least, that has not been the case for me. It is a daily grind to keep this reality in the front of my mind. To welcome the moments of peace and health and relish in the calm of that respite while recognizing that I was only truly guaranteed that moment.

One of my grandma's and mom's favorite quotes is, "This too shall pass." This became a mantra of mine in my quest for increasing sfumato in my life. Today, I feel like I can go and be a fully participating member of my family and feel actual joy. *This too shall pass.* Today, I feel I cannot get out of bed, my ears are ringing, and I feel hopeless and scared. *This too shall pass.* On my not-so-good days, I would think, *Okay, but WHEN!?* On a good day, I would rather not think about it. But over time, I learned it was important, so when the calm did pass, I didn't feel as if the rug had been pulled out from underneath me, leaving me lying on my butt and wondering what had happened.

Another mantra had been taped on my refrigerator growing up. It was another of my mom and dad's favorite quotes, "There is only a problem when there is a gap between expectation and reality." That problematic gap is what James Stockdale was referring to when he spoke about surviving a POW camp. You can't survive years of POW imprisonment if that gap is too large. One can't survive healing a medication injury, a medication discontinuation, or a benzo withdrawal if the gap is too wide, either. So, we need to work to close that gap and say to ourselves, *One day, I will be okay. Today might not be that day. Next month may not be the month, but one day. And for now, right now, I need to focus on what is in front of me at this moment and gather and implement the best tools and strategies to make it through.*

Remember those signs I spoke about earlier? I sometimes wonder if the reason the concept of *sfumato* hit me so hard and so instantaneously became a part of my vocabulary back when I was 29 years old is because one day, I would need it as my bedrock, my foundation, and my salvation. Who knows? All I know is that it felt like *truth* then, and I know it to be truth now.

CHAPTER TWENTY-THREE

DON'T BE A BEAD COLLECTOR, BUILD A RECOVERY NECKLACE

"Some people want it to happen,
some wish it would happen, others make it happen."

- Michael Jordan

I was mid-way through my career. I had completed my master's program, a post-master's fellowship, and I was working on my PhD. Additionally, I was running around getting certified in just about anything under the sun a therapist can get certified in. And one day, my older brother said, "Jen, I think you've got what you need."

I was hurt at first and thought, *No, I am a lifelong learner. This is only going to help me and my clients.* But after a few days, I really let what he said sink in and got honest with myself. Yes, I value always learning and would never claim to be an *expert* on anything or anyone. That said, there was also some truth to the notion that I was becoming a bead collector.

This is a metaphor I use with my clients a lot. The ones who read all the books, go to all the workshops, take notes in our therapy sessions, and yet seem frustrated that they are not progressing as they would like. There I was and there they were gathering up all of the beads, but the more we gathered, the more they slipped through our hands and fell to the floor. In order to make use of all of the wonderful beads of knowledge we are gathering, we have to slow down and string the beads into something of use. Make a necklace or a bracelet. Otherwise, the precious beads will continue to fall and roll away or find themselves at the bottom of some old drawer, forgotten.

I have shared many of the beads I have collected along the way in the previous chapters. Information I had gathered in reading hundreds of recovery narratives, quotes from books, philosophical and psychological strategies, and life lessons. But the real work has been finding a way to stop collecting at some point, slow down, and realize maybe I had enough beads to build my own recovery necklace. This is easier said than done, especially for someone like me, who is a natural researcher. However, putting things into action often gets lost or delayed due to the paralysis of analysis. (Remember that book I was going to write years ago that never launched?) I had to stop looking things up, stop reading 400 articles on the nervous system, and start to put together a daily practice—a recovery necklace—that would actually move me out of my head and fully into my healing.

Even as I write this chapter, I can tell you this is still the hardest thing for me. One week, I implement prayer and mindfulness like a recovery ninja, only to let that fall to the wayside the next week when I implement a bit more exercise. Just like my symptoms come at me like a giant whack-a-mole, my response to my injury is often just as sporadic and unpredictable.

I am learning that the nervous system likes stability and predictability. Medication injuries have rung the bell, and it takes a lot of time, patience, and perseverance to hone a practice that allows it to calm down. We are starting from the point of instability. So, the more our system can count on the amount of sleep, exercise, types of food and supplementation, hydration, and levels of stress it may encounter, the better off we will be. Some of this we don't have ultimate control over, especially sleep and stress levels. However, by having a sleep hygiene routine from which we don't deviate, our systems will know it's time to unwind even if it doesn't allow sleep to come on many nights. And although we cannot control all the variables that create stress in our lives, we can, as discussed earlier, control our attitude and our commitment to self-care, setting appropriate limits, and prioritizing our health.

So, join me in gathering up all of our beads of wisdom and stringing them together into a practice and attitude that creates a strong and sturdy necklace of recovery and healing. This necklace can serve as our lifeline as we do what this journey and Claire Weekes have both asked of us—LET TIME PASS.

CHAPTER TWENTY-FOUR

SHAME

*"What we don't need in the midst
of struggle is shame for being human."*

- Brene Brown

B rene Brown defines shame as, "The intensely painful feeling or experience of believing that we are flawed and therefore unworthy of love and belonging. *I am bad* or *I am a mess.* The focus is on the self, not behavior, with the result that we feel alone. Shame is never known to lead to positive change." If you haven't read much of Brene, please be sure to check out her incredible writing and work on shame and vulnerability.

My shame in all of this has been a big one for me. My entire career and role in my family have been built on being stable, reliable, dependable, and someone who shows up. To get hit with an injury that has left me *anything but* these traits has left me feeling deep shame about my limitations. When I was first *floxed*, it was the shame of having this invisible syndrome of symptoms and feeling like I should be able to pull myself together, snap out of it, and get back in the game. This shame further intensified as I felt gaslit by the medical community, who said there was nothing wrong with me and I needed to address my new-found anxiety disorder. Again, I didn't know anxiety disorders caused spine burning, a sense that one's brain is melting, an inability to regulate temperature, and neuropathy, but *okay*. (A bit of sarcasm? A bit. I'm not angry any longer, just still in disbelief that this was how all of this was received.)

Years later, when I was re-injured and realized I could not simply walk off the benzodiazepine I had taken as prescribed, the shame returned. Here I was: a therapist working with my patients on skills to help them *not* rely on benzodiazepines and sleeping pills, and I was stuck. I had to do some deep soul searching, and I found that what was most helpful was to be as honest as I could with my clients. I hadn't done anything wrong. I wasn't a drug seeker. I had gotten snared by taking a med in the properly prescribed manner. It still took a long time for me not to beat myself up while feeling I should have known better. But shame, I found out, was too expensive a commodity, and I was now on a tight emotional budget. I simply could not afford it.

I don't remember the process of letting go of the shame, but that is exactly what has occurred. In fact, in its place has come a humility the likes I had never known in myself before. I don't fear what people will think of me, how they view me or my injury. I began to use it as a wonderful filter. People that were judgmental, unable to show up, upset that I was no longer able to show up as I once had, were simply too expensive. I couldn't afford them either, and I had to peacefully and lovingly let them go. I learned to become comfortable with being vulnerable.

Again, Brene has a great way of capturing this self-state; she describes vulnerability as "...having the courage to show up when you can't control the outcome."

I also realized that if I were going to try to use my situation to support others as well as advocate for informed consent and proper de-prescribing protocol, I would need to let go of the shame to share my story with full transparency. On a more personal level, I had to learn to become okay going to family dinners and celebrations knowing that I would need to bring my own food, might need to step into a quiet room for a half-hour to avoid sensory overload, and might even need to leave if things started to feel too much for me. I am still working to challenge myself on good days and weeks to meet a friend out for lunch or dinner knowing it may prove to be too much, and I might need to duck out early.

As stated earlier in this book, we are not in full control of this healing process. But we can assist our nervous systems that are working so hard to heal for us by letting go of the weight of shame and embracing our vulnerability, humility, and self-compassion.

CHAPTER TWENTY-FIVE
ANGER AT PEOPLE WHO "DON'T GET IT"

"For every minute you remain angry,
you give up sixty seconds of peace of mind."

- Ralph Waldo Emerson

I think anyone who has experienced a significant illness, death, divorce, or trauma of other sorts can relate to the adage, "You find out who your friends are." As I stated earlier, as painful as it is, our struggle quickly separates those that will stay and those who, for many reasons, just can't. Initially, I had a lot of anger at doctors, friends, and loved ones who I felt didn't really work to understand what I was going through. It was easy to fall into some self-pity and to feel their absence as judgment.

Again, anger is expensive, and I am on a tight budget. There is just no healthy, sustainable way to hang onto it for long without it interfering in our healing process. I began to recognize the power of forgiveness. Instead of feeling like a victim, I realized there was a lot of agency and power in radically accepting people's varied responses and forgiving them if they could not show up for me. This is true of the doctors along the way that made me feel crazy and folks along the way that just didn't have much to offer. I also had and have to own that I am not the easiest person to offer help. I tend to clam up rather than ask for help and go inside myself rather than share what I am going through. So, part of my work has been recognizing my part in not being a great repository for what folks might have to offer. This is still a huge learning curve for me.

I believe part of the larger issue stems from what is ingrained in us. Look at the way we handle bereavement in our culture. Three days off from work max in most places. The casseroles come in for a few days, and then a week or so later, life has moved on. During those years I worked in hospice, we sent volunteers out for sometimes over a year to visit with families after their loved one had died. The casseroles had long stopped arriving, and the push for them to return to work, their lives, and their roles often brought about a sense of isolation, anxiety, and depression that was crushing.

It's the same for chronic or long-term illnesses. If I had a nickel for every time someone asked me, "Don't they have a medication to help you?" I would be a rich woman. I'm not sure about the rest of the world, but I know here in the U.S.A., we want a quick fix. We can't stand to watch people we care about in long-term suffering. It also brings up a fear that it could happen to us. For example, after three big family losses in a short period of time, my mom was told by a friend, "I don't want to get too close in case your bad luck is contagious."

I have another friend suffering from tremendous burnout in her career. If she lived in Amsterdam, she could go to the doctor, and if clinically warranted, the doctor would write a note to her employer saying she suffered from *burnout* and needs a month off to recuperate. Here in the States, we are given a handful of psychiatric diagnoses, usually with accompanying medications followed by a deep shame that we are now deemed either short-term or long-term *disabled*. That's if you work for a company that even offers those benefits. For most, there is simply no option other than to leave your work position or stay and push through your emotional and physical duress and stress.

All of this is to say that we are not a culture with much patience or empathy for vulnerability, illness, or loss. So, it only makes sense that the people that make up that culture often share that same perspective and struggle to really hang in there long-term with people as they grapple with their ailment or situation. I am not saying I am okay with this. I am simply saying that when put in perspective, I was able to shift my expectations. It also made me really focus my energy on gratitude for those that could stand by and show up.

I know this has changed me fundamentally. I would like to believe I was a friend or loved one who always showed up. I know it was always a value of mine, and I tried to show up well and often, but I also know there were times I fell off along the way. I wasn't always the most reliable friend. I now know better. I also know I can't have 30 friends and think I can show up for them through thick and thin. I have an immediate family of nearly 25 people. I have to be very thoughtful about where I put my energy outside of that family system. Again, it's all *mentalomics*. I can't afford shame. I can't afford anger or resentment. And I don't have endless psychic or empathic energy to expend. Therefore, if someone can only afford to call and check in with me once a month, I appreciate that. If they can't for various reasons, then I work to accept this and not see it as a personal rejection or failure on either my part or theirs.

Chapter Twenty-Six
Too Much Time on the Internet

"Well, there's another five hours
of my life I'll never get back!"

- Me

Okay, so this is a tricky subject. I hate to say stay off the web and the sites. Had I not found Benzo Buddies and several Facebook support groups, I would have had no idea what was happening to me in episode two of my injury. In this group, I learned how to taper off the benzodiazepine properly, found normalization of my wide array of scary symptoms, and met a few dear friends that I continue to be in daily contact with as I navigate this journey. These sites all became very important sources of information, data, support, and amazing stories of success and recovery that were incredibly helpful and inspiring.

However, I quickly found that too much of anything is typically not good for us. This certainly proved to be the case with going on the forums and sites. On bad days, I would find myself reading horror story after horror story and chasing all of my symptoms into the darkest and scariest of rabbit holes. The sites, especially the success stories, can inspire hope, but as I have said in many ways throughout this book, we get good at what we practice. It matters what we feed our minds. When our minds and central nervous systems are injured, what we feed ourselves becomes even more critical. In this process, we are so much more sensitive and suggestible. A scary story that some random person shares can twist, turn, and take root in our psyches bringing forth shock waves of terror and anxiety.

All of us are unique individuals living our own lives, and this is incredibly true in our recovery. What works for one may not work for another and vice versa. Therefore, the stories people share on the sites can be informative about their own experiences but not necessarily be helpful to ours. That said, sometimes, there are patterns of experiences. While this pattern may not hold true in your own recovery process, they can be helpful to understand. For example, many folks who incur an antibiotic injury, or even on the gabapentin sites, sing the praises of taking magnesium supplements to aid in recovery. However, on the sites for people in benzodiazepine withdrawal, magnesium is controversial as it can interface with the GABA-A receptor and can create huge problems for some people in their taper and recovery process. This doesn't mean one shouldn't take magnesium, but it provides a series of anecdotal data points to help you decide about trying it. This is just one example of how the sites can be both useful and also lead to further confusion and struggle as we try to apply what worked for one individual to our unique situation, hoping for a similar, positive outcome.

For many people, the sites can be triggering and overwhelming. Others view them as their lifeline in the recovery process. I land somewhere in the middle. Ultimately, I'm incredibly grateful for them. However, I need to manage the investment of time and mental energy I spend on the sites to preserve my own sense of calm and healing.

One thing that I found lifesaving in this process was to stop reading about antibiotics, med injuries, or benzodiazepines, and when I could, pick up a book about *anything* but these topics. I found I could really only concentrate on fiction novels between the hours of 10:00 p.m. and 1:00 a.m., so it was during those hours that I would either read or write. Over the course of this past summer, I read all of Elin Hilderbrand's novels, and my mind could escape its torment for a few hours and escape to Nantucket or St. John with a host of lively characters. I also returned to my entire childhood collection of Judy Blume books and allowed myself to resort back to a more innocent time in life when medications and health concerns were far from my young mind. I loved hanging back out with Margaret, SuperFudge, Blubber, and Deenie and losing myself in their pre-teenage angst, humor, and antics.

Another book I found and re-read was the book *Breakfast with Buddha* by Roland Merullo. I had read it years before, but one day, as I was passing by my bookshelf, there was a book sticking out at a strange angle. I found it odd as I hadn't used that particular shelf in months, but as I went to straighten it, I pulled it out. It was Merullo's book. I was having a particularly bad few days, had spent way too much time on the sites, and was feeling hopeless and scared. My faith in myself and the world felt weary. I devoured the book that night, looked up the author, found an email address, and decided to write him a thank-you note. I told him I had been sick, re-read the book, and felt moved and encouraged by the story. The *next day* I had an email back from Roland, and I got goosebumps as I felt some of my trust and love of humanity restored. I realized we aren't so separate and that by putting my attention on something outside of my symptoms for just a little while, I had tapped into a needed part of myself and made a connection with a beautiful human being. Roland ended up mailing me a copy of another book he had written and offered his prayers and support.

It was a great reminder that there is a whole world outside of my four walls of suffering. While the groups and sites can be enormously helpful, it is important to venture out and beyond every once in a while to be reminded of this fact.

Chapter Twenty-Seven

Idle Time

"The bad news is time flies.
The good news is you're the pilot."

- Michael Altshuler

The chapter on time spent online is a nice segue into a discussion about idle time. This is another topic that is challenging for me. There have been many days, even weeks, where it would have been physically or mentally impossible to maintain a daily task or routine. However, on days or times when there was even a shard of me that felt intact, I felt it was critical to try to engage my life on some level.

On my better days, I could show up for my family, work on writing this book, or try out other creative endeavors. Over time, I found that I did better if I had some sort of schedule, even on my bad days. Even if it was just 1) get up, 2) eat breakfast, 3) reach out to one person, 4) get out of the house for at least 20 minutes, 5) think about or do something for someone else (send a nice text, email, or phone call).

I remember one day in particular when I was feeling down and struggling. I knew I needed to find *Aunt Jen*. My most favorite two words on the planet. The words that have always offered me my greatest purpose. I knew I didn't have much in the proverbial tank, but I left my home and got in the car, drove to Crave cupcakes, bought cupcakes for my six nieces and nephews who lived nearby and dropped them off at their respective homes. It was imperative that I tap into this beloved role and not allow my injury or illness to rob me of it any more than it had. I didn't feel great doing it, but it gave me something to do that mattered to me. A few months ago, when my symptoms had worsened and I could not drive, I decided to take my typical one hour of relief each night and write a letter of gratitude to people that I love. I couldn't drop off cupcakes, but I could find some way to step outside of my pain for a moment.

Idle time in this process can be dangerous. Hear me when I say I am not advocating for keeping yourself busy as a means to avoid your situation. I am referring to the fact that a minute in this process can feel like a week if we aren't careful. Days can run together, and I often feel like I am reliving Groundhog Day by waking up each morning to another version of hell. Idle time can lock me in my head with thoughts that are disturbing and unhealthy. Believe me, in this process, it often appears I am in idle time. I do a lot of praying, meditating, resting, deep breathing, and grounding and centering myself. But I don't consider that idle time. Idle time for me often takes the form of going on the forums and sites and losing myself for hours in the horror of others' experiences. Idle time can sometimes take the form of getting locked in my head and getting lost in the *if onlys* and *what ifs?*

Remember, *mentalomics* is the name of the game. And idle time, at least for me, is often an investment that yields no return and might even create a deficit in the economy of myself and my health.

CHAPTER TWENTY-EIGHT

BELIEVING THE LIE OF THE HOLE

"There are things known and there are things unknown, and in between are the doors of perception."

- Aldous Huxley

In my clinical practice, I would often talk with my clients about the problematic dynamic that I referred to as the *lie of the hole*. Basically, this is something that can and often does happen to the healthiest of us. However, it can be more prevalent and intense when we get hooked by our thoughts or negative feelings.

Let me offer up an example. I was working with a woman struggling off and on with bouts of depression and agitation. She didn't meet the full criteria for major depressive disorder. Over time we tracked the cycle of her mood to a near monthly "girls night out" in which she drank too much, rarely ate, and got little to no sleep. However, prior to our making this realization, every month or so, I would get a call outside of our typical weekly session in which my client was distressed, felt certain her husband was no longer attracted to her, was paranoid he might be having an affair and would become so dysregulated that she would threaten to leave him.

After a few days, she would come in or call and say things like, "All is well. I am not leaving him. I don't know what was wrong with me, but I adore him, and he just wrote me the most loving card and left it for me with tickets to see my favorite band." We explored how month after month of having days of intense distrust, insecurity, and highly reactive behavior would eventually drive the calmest, most understanding husband to the brink of exhaustion and frustration. I told her to imagine that she had fallen into a hole. In that hole, all that she knew before was lost to her. She couldn't remember the light, the solid ground, the comforts of life. All she could feel was despair, distrust, fear, and hopelessness.

We agreed—*the hole lies.* For 98% of the month, she never doubted her husband's loyalty or motives. But in the hole, she was certain that her suspicious and distrusting thoughts and feelings were completely true and valid. We decided to write a letter that she would keep in her lockbox, and the next time she felt those feelings reappear, she was to reach in and grab and read the letter. The letter was a letter to herself that basically read:

"Dear _____,

Yep, here we are again, my dear. We've slipped back into our hole. This hole will tell you that your husband is cheating on you, that he is a liar, and that you are being manipulated. The hole will make you feel less than, and you will begin to engage in self-destructive behaviors to punish both yourself and him. These are not truths, and in about 72 hours, a giant spotlight will shine down into this hole and eradicate all of these thoughts and feelings that right now you are convinced are truth. Let's not do this. If in five days, you still think or feel this way, then we think about whether or not to act on them."

Not once did she feel or think the thoughts five days later, and over time, she stopped giving them much mind at all when they would arise. Over time, as I said, we were able to link them to a particular external factor and recognize that she, like most of us, has times that are more vulnerable than others. We need to not let the holes we fall into take hold of our hearts and minds, convincing us that the darkness holds the truth.

I have found this to be very important in my process of recovery as well. A lot of people in the benzo world talk about the *benzo lie*. The *benzo brain* often creates highly disturbing thoughts and feelings that are experienced as truths and facts, thus increasing our fear and dread that the world is scary or dangerous. I had this same experience when I was *floxed* back in 2016. My brain would play tricks on me. One hour, I could be having a nice conversation with a friend only to find myself three hours later convinced that I was a burden, was losing my mind, and going to lose all of my relationships.

Just like my client, it is imperative that we don't believe the *lie of the hole* of medication injury. Some of those lies are: *I am going to lose my mind. I am never going to get better. I have a new symptom that must mean I am getting worse. Everyone is tired of me. I am such a burden. I just need to get reassurance one more time (for the hundredth time today) that I am going to be okay because I am not going to be okay. I*

am unique, and no one is as bad off as I am. I must have done some-
thing to deserve or create this... I could keep going. The lies are
endless, and they can be torturous.

Most of us with medication injuries develop *sticky mind,*
where we have difficulty relinquishing distressing thoughts. I've
found it critical that I learn to recognize the *lie of the hole* for what
it is and learn how to navigate my way out of the hole to keep
the lies from driving me crazy.

As I stated earlier, one of the assumptions I tend to make
over and over again in this process is that one bad day is an in-
dicator of a series of days or that things are taking a turn for the
worst. Just as problematic at times was the assumption that a
good day meant I was taking a turn for the better only to be hit
with symptoms and find myself falling back into despair and
disillusionment.

Again, this is where using the ideas in the Stockdale Paradox
becomes our saving grace. *I know I will be okay one day. Today isn't*
that day. Tomorrow, next week, or next month might not be either. But
one day. In the meantime, let me buckle up and ride out this fresh hell I
am in right now. A bad day is just what it is. A good day is just
what it is. There are no assumptions to be made or promises to
be believed in this non-linear process. While that might be mad-
dening to accept, I can promise you it is infinitely more of a
mind screw to believe that one hour, one symptom, one thing
can predict another. I am learning—and believe me, I am a terrible student—that we have to just be where we are and work to
accept whatever window or wave we might be experiencing. We

cannot believe the lie of the hole that these med injuries carve out in our psyches.

CHAPTER TWENTY-NINE

COMPARING MYSELF TO OTHERS

"The tip of the neighbor's iceberg often looks very nice."

- Roy A. Ngansop

O h man, this is a tough one. I can't tell you how many hours have been clocked compulsively checking my symptoms against the symptoms of other people. I would look up their stories and their symptoms and then think, *But wait, they are four years older than me. They tapered faster. They are not on any other meds. They didn't eat as clean as I do. They weren't floxed before starting on a benzo. They don't seem to be as sensitive as me...* on and on. I lost hundreds of hours both wanting to find my story in the story of someone else (but only one who had a successful ending) or to absolutely see how my story was unique and no one was as bad as me.

It's completely natural to do this, but time and time again, this only offered a temporary reprieve from my anxiety. I now have a commitment with my trauma triplets that should I want to *go trolling the stories* online, I am to reach out to them first. They serve as my first line of accountability towards stopping this loop that tends to only lead to further fear and angst.

Reading success stories was helpful and useful at times. But often, I was looking for myself in these stories and comparing pain. This is not helpful. In fact, it often made things much worse. The worst kind of pain is our own. Period.

Even with my friends in this process, I have to be careful not to get mired down in comparison. *They are so much further along than me. They are doing so much better than me...* again, not helpful. For me, it has only been hurtful. While we don't want to be alone in this process, the reality is that there is no one with your exact experience, symptoms, or recovery process. Thus, spending hours trying to find it in someone else or comparing your pain to their own is a waste of time and energy. (And remember, we are on a tight budget when it comes to energy.)

CHAPTER THIRTY

CHOOSE WELL AND BE GENTLE
WITH YOURSELF AND OTHERS

"Nothing is so strong as gentleness,
nothing so gentle as real strength."

- Saint Francis de Sales

nother thing that has been incredibly unhelpful to me has been the times when I put this sacred story and journey into the hands of the wrong people. There are many people who, for whatever reason, cannot join us on this journey. I learned this the hard way a few times, but I have slowly figured out this narrative is my own. It's not a pretty, fun, and enjoyable narrative to share or to hear, but it is mine.

Once I started to have some regard and compassion for myself and my experience, it was clear that how and with whom I chose to share my story needed to come from the same place of regard and compassion.

Along with this came the realization that I didn't have to hold a grudge towards those that couldn't or didn't want to hear. I could offer them compassion and regard as well. But I needed to use my theory of *mentalomics* and be incredibly discerning regarding who I would open up to and let in.

For example, I found myself wanting to explain my situation to any doctor that I have seen over these years. There have been one or two that really pulled up a chair, listened, and seemed genuinely interested. But there were also a few who never even made eye contact, never slowed down, or merely feigned concern or interest. So, I never stopped trying, but when I realized that I didn't have their ear, I learned to protect myself. This is a very important part of my experience.

With regard to friends and loved ones, this discernment and self-protection can feel more isolating and painful. Look, it is not easy to have a front-row seat for this kind of suffering. Some can stay with us, and some have to go. Some can stay for a while but may need to duck out, catch their breath, and then return. Some seem to be able to ride it out along with us all the way through.

And sometimes, the folks that maybe can't hear or stay in the beginning may enter at a different phase of our recovery. I have found that some people who couldn't show up well in the beginning became great supporters and allies later on in my journey. Some that showed interest and concern in the beginning just kind of moved away the further and longer the injury stuck around.

I found it important to protect my story and be very discerning in choosing whom, how, and when to share it. Most of all, I needed grace to permeate this process for myself and those I cared about, both those that could stick around and those that just couldn't for whatever reason.

I have found that my sense of pride and any modesty I had prior to this process no longer exists. That said, another way we need to *choose wisely* is how much information we share. I can pick up the phone with my trauma triplets and tell them all about my poop, my ureter burning, and hear about their various aches and pains. I can reach out to Geraldine and share an intrusive, disturbing thought. I have been on the phone with a friend as we peed on sticks to ensure we hadn't developed a UTI, and our biggest fear was that we might need an antibiotic (a huge fear in the world of the CNS compromised).

But the reality is most of the world does not want to hear about the fact that I can hear my heartbeat in my head, feel my spine dance, hear things being said three rooms away, how my bowels are working, what my menstrual cycles are like, if I was able to shower that day, my fear of bananas, or any number of bizarre things I am now hyperaware of and feel the need to share.

Humor and humility replaced modesty and shame for me. These were positive replacements; however, they can sometimes leave me with no filter leading me to disclose a litany of wacky symptoms and experiences that very few people want to be privy to.

CHAPTER THIRTY-ONE

HUMOR

*"There is a fine line that separates laughter and pain,
comedy and tragedy, humor and hurt."*

- Erma Bombeck

I contemplated leaving this chapter blank.

But the reality is that as dark and scary and painful as med injuries are, I had to find shreds of humor in it. First of all, finding some humor is a reminder that all is not lost. It's like the idea that a person worrying they might be psychotic most certainly isn't psychotic. Or a person who worries they are narcissistic typically is not a raging narcissist. When I can manage just a slight distance from my suffering and allow a bit of light and humor to pervade, I am no longer just a bag of skin and bones shuffling through a hellish experience.

Along the way, I have belly laughed about my friend's fear of bananas. I have laughed at myself as I peed on the seventh home test strip, terrified it might show a UTI, and as I went and had three COVID tests in two weeks out of pure fear that I had developed the virus (despite never leaving my home and being around no one for months on end). My trauma triplets and I have, in our darkest times, been able to laugh at ourselves and each other as we realize that at any other time in our lives, we would not be discussing the color of our poop, a tiny growth on our shin, or why I had suddenly developed a fear of documentaries and Pixar movies.

I am not f#*ked up. This is a f#*ked up process, and if I don't let humor creep in, I will go down and stay down.

CHAPTER THIRTY-TWO

BECOMING A PERSON OF RECORD

"True freedom is the capacity for acting according to one's true character, to be altogether one's self, to be self-determined and not subject to outside coercion."

- Corliss Lamont

A few years ago, I began writing a book called *Raising a Person of Record: Effective Parenting in an Anxious World*. As I said earlier, I don't believe in accidents. For some reason, it wasn't time for that book to be birthed by me. I now think I have some understanding as to why. The concept I came up with—*person of record*—was one I could intellectually describe. But I now know that it was not a fully lived experience of my own. Therefore, any writing about it would be intellectual and re-moved at best.

As I mentioned at the beginning of this book, each day I deepen my awareness that this is a process of transformation and social/emotional/physical/spiritual alchemy. I am already changed for the better, and I believe through this highly painful process, I will emerge my best self. I will emerge a person of record. What do I mean by a "person of record?" Here are just a few of the traits:

1. They have a sense of integrity—I am not speaking about morality here but more in the sense of the word integrous—a sense of wholeness, a coherent sense of self. *I'm going to be okay because I take me wherever I go, and I know myself.* People of record know where they end and others begin. Thus, they tend to be good at implementing and holding healthy boundaries and limits.

2. In knowing themselves, they are good at accepting their limitations and recognizing their strengths.

3. They are able to mentalize with relative consistency.

4. They are reliable and consistent.

5. They have a strong sense of personal accountability.

6. They have integrity with their speech. They say what they mean, and they mean what they say.

7. They do not externalize blame or lead with judgment or assumption to feel better.

8. They employ what I call the five Cs: calm, clear, curious, compassionate, and contained.

9. They understand their own *mentalomics*.

10. They operate at the speed of wisdom.

11. They tend to keep their heads up and eyes open. They don't walk or look away in the face of a challenge.

12. They tend to understand that they were not promised that life was meant to be easy, and they have developed a mental resilience to *stay* in the wake of discomfort or distress.

13. They do not expend a great deal of energy on things that they do not have control over. Remember the *Serenity Prayer*–courage, strength, and wisdom.

14. They tend to come from an abundance model versus a scarcity model. They feel there is more than enough to go around, and thus, they are collaborative and encouraging rather than competitive and envious.

I never finished the book. As I said, it has just been in the last few months that I have realized why. I wasn't ready to finish it. Clinically, I could understand these self traits. I could see how we could work as parents, teachers, and clinicians to help instill them in our children, students, and clients to help them become strong yet flexible selves. Healthy selves. But in my life lived, I did not know these traits consistently or intimately. I needed to become a person of record. Then, and only then, would my work and writing be authentic and helpful.

This painful injury has brought me to the brink. The brink of my sanity, my sense of myself, my understanding of what really matters, and even at moments, to the brink of my own existence as I know it. This process has the power to carve me into the self I have always had the potential to be—if I can remain vertical, breathing, and faithful long enough to allow it. I pray that I can find it within myself to hang on and allow the healing to happen. I believe I will emerge from what appears to be the wreckage of my life with a renewed sense of health, faith, courage, and wisdom. Through this process of alchemy, I aim to intimately know what it means to be a person of record, and I am already working on finishing writing the book I began so many years ago.

CHAPTER THIRTY-THREE

HEALING HURTS

"The wound is the place where the light enters you."

- Rumi

I'll end on a positive note. I can't tell you the number of times along the way I have asked myself and others the questions, *Am I healing as I taper off this medication? Can I heal from benzos if I am on any other medication?* Or *Is healing possible with so much damage from being floxed and then the on and off again of these meds?*

I asked this in my conversations with Chris, Christy, Baylissa, Geraldine, and Jennifer—all warriors and past fellow inmates of this particular brand of hell. All of them said, "Yes." However, I realized that until I believed, *Yes, I am healing,* it didn't matter how much reinforcement I called in.

When I shattered my elbow, it hurt like hell for months as it healed. Healing hurts. Now I work very hard to remember, especially on days when I feel bombarded with symptoms, *This is my brain and my central nervous system trying to heal me.* Believe me, on a bad day, this is a very, very hard sell. However, if I can get just a slight crack of light in, I can feel the power of those words at work. Every moment of every day, I am healing.

As I said before, it is non-linear. It is unpredictable. But whether it's a good day or a day riddled with symptoms, my body is working on my behalf. Each day if I feed it well, try to rest it, walk it, let it fully breathe, and allow time to pass when I feel distraught, I know I am one step closer to the ecstasy I believe I will one day feel on the other side. I am not alone in this. This is what I have been given to walk through. I didn't ask for this, and it is not something I would wish on my least favorite person. But it is my lot, my experience to have. My *fati to amor*. And we ARE healing.

I'll end with one of my favorite quotes from Michael Singer, "Everything will be okay when I am okay with everything." When I read this quote a few years back, I knew I was in trouble. I got goosebumps, which meant it resonated as truth for me. Just like the word *sfumato*, this also meant that it would most likely show back up in my life and have some significance. Little did I know that I would be given the ultimate test just months later—how could I possibly get "okay" with this? Being okay with this injury and recovery process doesn't mean I am enjoying it. It simply means coming to terms that this is my reality. The more I resist my reality, the more it will punch back. So, let's all lean in, accept, learn, have faith, hold ourselves gentle and tight, and know that everything will be okay (one day).

FAITH, REVISITED:
THE WAITING ROOM

This book wasn't originally called *The Waiting Room*. It was called *Flox My Life: When Good Meds Turn Bad*. I had finished writing it, had sent it to a few trusted people, including my brother, Rhys, for editing, and was looking to move ahead towards the process of publication. I had found a small publishing house that showed interest, and all I had to do was hit send. I couldn't. I stared at it for days, wondering why suddenly I couldn't touch it, had no desire to try to get it published, and felt ripples of fear and dread when I thought about doing so.

Just days after finishing it, I entered into the worst wave I have encountered since entering withdrawal. Remember when med injury recovery affects our nervous system, the non-linear healing experiences are often referred to as *windows* (good moments) and *waves* (not so good moments). For me, the terms were highly relevant to my personal experience of feeling a few hours or maybe, if lucky, a few days where I felt joy, peace, and a sense of myself. In my windows, I could feel the deep love for my family and friends and could dream again of a life where I could get up in the morning and go for a walk; talk to a few clients; or take my beloved nieces and nephews for candy, ice cream, or out for dinner. But damn, those waves. Just as my

191

head was above the surf and I could see a way through, inevitably, a wave of the most intense mental and physical anguish would crash over me, sending me and my smile and dreams scraping against the bottom of the sea, disoriented, disappointed and terrified. Unfortunately, this wave began slowly building months ago and has been more like a *crash* than a wave.

One evening, as I sat in bed working on a latch hook rug of a panda... Wait, let me stop here. Yes, I started to do latch hook rugs as a way to try to distract myself from myself. I am not creative. I cannot cook, draw, sing, crochet, sew, or paint. Apparently, I cannot latch hook, either. The panda was my first, and it was god-awful. As ugly as it was, when I called Mop (nickname for my niece Meghan) at Notre Dame and told her I was making it for her dorm room, she teared up. Meghan is not one for a lot of tears, so I believe she deeply understood the tenuous road I was walking if I was sitting in my apartment latch hooking a panda bear.

Anyway, one night amidst this wave, while *Flox My Life* sat on my computer screen staring at me as I felt unable to send it off, I turned on an audible book by Max Lucado. The narrator began reading a chapter, and it was about being in God's waiting room. I set my latch hook aside and stared at my phone. It was as if Max was speaking directly to me. He told the story of Joseph and his long, painful yet faithful wait for God. I realized this was what I needed to hear. Earlier in the day, I had a few hours where the mental weight of my situation overwhelmed me. I doubted I could do it much longer. How could I continue on? And how long would it take until I was healed? Would I heal? But those words spoke directly to my heart.

Then as synchronicity would have it, a beloved friend of mine sent me another small book by Max Lucado and his daughter. In the book, I learned of the story of Joshua. God instructed Joshua to, along with his army, receive (not take over) the city of Jericho. But Jericho was a city surrounded by two concentric 40-foot-high stone walls, and the evils that took place within those walls were known to many. God sent him on his way and instructed him on how to penetrate this city that had been impenetrable until then. Joshua went back to his army and told them of their mission, and they yelled and cheered, excited to take their axes to the stone walls, their swords to the fight. Then Joshua explained that was not the plan. The plan was to be led by seven priests, the ark of the covenant, and to march silently while the priests sounded a ram's horn. I am sure the troops thought Joshua was nuts but complied. They walked silently around the walls of that city for seven days, not understanding their mission nor the purpose of what they were being asked. On the seventh day, Joshua said, "Scream out," and they did. The walls collapsed and fell to the ground.

My health situation, my iatrogenic central nervous system injury, is my Jericho. My healing and this process is not in my time frame. If Joshua's troops had bailed on day six, they wouldn't have gained their city on day seven. Had Joseph given up on year 12, he would not have been brought to Pharaoh and freed from imprisonment. If Chris Paige had given up at year three from his constant battle with akathisia, he would never be back in his career helping so many others heal from med injuries. If my grandma had given up and given in to her abuse, she would not have escaped rural Georgia with my mom, and I would not be here telling this story. I am in God's waiting room. While I am in this waiting room, there are things I can do, beliefs I can change, attitudes I can shift to help me along and hopefully give meaning to this hellish journey. Then when I am called out of the waiting room, I will emerge a stronger, more resilient, and healthier version of myself than when I went in. The title *Flox My Life*, in retrospect, sounds angry and fatalistic. *The Waiting Room* to me, represents faith, endurance, "smart effort," and hope. I do not know how long the wait will be, but I know with all of my heart, mind, and soul that it will be worth it. Who knows if I have lapped Jericho twice or six times? Only time will tell. Until then, I hold firmly to the notion that *this too shall pass*.

ACKNOWLEDGMENTS

There are so many people that I quite literally owe my life to in this process that it's hard to know where to begin.

To Mom and Dad: I am 51 years old and the tables have not turned. You are still my role models, my rock, my safe place to land. When the ground beneath me gave out, you never questioned, judged, or left me. You have been right by my side in the hardest time of my life, and I would never be able to capture in words the love and respect I have for you both. Thank you for seeing me during times when I couldn't even recognize myself. You taught me that with love, there is always room. No one is left behind with the two of you at the helm. I love you.

To my best friend, my partner in life, and the best egg I know: Shawnie. You have stood by me during my absolute darkest moments. Your selflessness inspires me, and your earnestness, strength, and quirkiness never cease to amaze and amuse me. Thank you for stepping up and in at a time when most people would have turned to run. I love you!

To "my ten:" On November 20, 2000, the best part of me was born. I became "Aunt Jen" for the first time. You all have given me purpose, direction, and a love I had never known existed inside of me. Meghan, Jack, Ryan, Austin, Aiden, Abby, Rhys,

Mary, Riley, and Olivia—you are my "why" and my "how."

To my family: Jeff, Allison, Kevin, Wendy, Rhys, Amy, Paula, Dustin, Hayden, and Lucia—your love and acceptance have offered and continue to offer me a safe space to heal and grow. I love you!

To my pups, Attie and Bailey: You have literally been by my side and made sure I was never alone even in my darkest moments. You are the best fur babies anyone could ask for. I love you!

To Sandra Lopez: You have been my port in the storm. You are the most amazing therapist and God must have known what lay ahead for me when he brought us together. I can't imagine having to do this without you.

To Geraldine Burns: You are one of the true matriarchs of the benzo awareness movement. More importantly, you are my dear friend and one of the most generous people I have ever encountered.

To Elizabeth and Lisa, my triplets: From laughing until we cried about the absurdities of our situations to a silent, reverential "I am here" when the pain was just too great—I am so blessed to have found you both.

To Bob and Debbie, Art and Debbie, Dan, Lisa, Tresa, Debbie, Cara, Shannon, Sarah, Elise, Ben, Blake, Diana, Jim, Cheryl, Meghan, Marki, Cynthia M., Kim, Rachel, Barbara, Chris Paige, Christy Huff, Nicole Lamberson, David Powers, Jennifer Leigh, Jimmy, Laura, Cynthia P., Jen, Natalie, Sofia, Lisa, Katie, Marilee, Michelle, Trina, Diane, Ken, Justin, Baylissa, Taylor,

Lori, Stephanie and Scott, Kathy, Weezer, Alex and Medley, Jackie, Deanna, Snuffy, and so many others: You have been with me in various ways along this path. Whether you were reaching out a hand for me, I for you, sitting side by side in the muck, or you simply held a placard for me in your life knowing I would and WILL one day return better than ever, I am forever grateful.

To Dr. Norma Clarke: Thank you for not giving up on me even when we didn't know which way to turn. You didn't abandon ship, and I have learned with certain med injuries and benzo withdrawal, sometimes that is the only and the best thing a doctor can offer you.

To Dr. Blackmon: Internists like you are a gem. Thank you for believing me. Thank you for not being one in a list of many who wrote me off and told me it was all in my head. I was lost that day that you sat and spent NINETY minutes with me, and I left your office feeling sane and seen.

To Robert Henry and Robin Locke Monda: Thank you for your professionalism and partnership in helping me get this book written, covered, and launched!

To my beloved clients: It was one of the hardest things in my life to close down my practice and walk away from you. Each of you inspired me with your vulnerability, your strength, and your kindness. I have loved being a therapist, and I always walked away feeling I had gained more than I had given. I hope you are all on a healing path and know that you deserve great things.

To Grandma Paula: You may have left this world 34 years ago, but you are in my heart and mind as if I just got back from one of "our weeks" together. Thank you for sending off a flare and a sign to remind me to "keep going." I know it's you.

To God: I have had a friendship with you for a long time. I have been angry with you at moments along the way, but I also know that you granted me this time slot for a reason. I hope I am doing it justice, Lord.

REFERENCE/READING LIST

Disclaimer: Any and all of these resources are simply publications, organization, websites, videos, and people that I have found helpful in my process. This list is intended for informational and educational purposes only, not to be used or seen as prescriptive advice or meant to replace recommendations/referrals offered to you by your own clinical/medical support team.

- *The Benzodiazepine Crisis: The Ramifications from an Overused Drug Class* edited by S. Wright, et.al.

- *Drug Dealer, MD: How Doctors Were Duped, Patients got Hooked, and Why It's So Hard to Stop* by Dr. Anna Lembke

- *The Benzo Book* by Jack Hobson-Dupont

- *Recovery and Renewal* by Baylissa Frederick

- *Hope and Healing for your Nerves* by Dr. Claire Weekes (all of her books are wonderful and she narrates many of them herself on Audible)

- *Seeds of Hope* by Jocelyn Pederson

- *Blood Orange Night: My Journey of Madness* by Melissa Bond

- *The Anxious Truth* by Drew Insalata

- *Man's Search for Meaning* by Viktor Frankl

- *The Untethered Soul* by Mickey Singer

- *The Surrender Experiment* by Mickey Singer

- *Stillness is the Key* by Ryan Holiday

- *The Obstacle is the Way* by Ryan Holiday

- *Courage is Calling* by Ryan Holiday

- *Meditations* by Marcus Aurelius

- *DARE* by Barry McDonagh

- All of Max Lucado's books (especially loved *Traveling Light* and *Anxious for Nothing*)

- *He Fights for You* by Max and Andrea Lucado

- *Overcoming Intrusive Thoughts* by Sally Winston and Martin Seif

- *Needing to Know for Sure* by Martin Seif and Sally Winston

- *Overcoming Anticipatory Anxiety* by Martin Seif and Sally Winston

- *Self-Compassion: The Proven Power of Being Kind to Yourself* by Kristin Neff

- *The Anxious Truth* by Drew Linsalata

- *An Anxiety Story* by Drew Linsalata

- *Death Grip: A Climbers Escape from Benzo Madness* by Matt Samet

- *At Last a Life* by Paul David

- All of Brene Brown's books

- All of Pema Chodron's books

- *The Biology of Belief* by Bruce Lipton, PhD

Other Resources

(certainly not exhaustive, but a good start)

- *The Benzo Information Coalition*

- *Mad in America* – blogs and articles regarding psychotropic issues/injuries

- *The Inner Compass Initiative* and *The Withdrawal Project* on Facebook (great interviews regarding withdrawal from psychotropic meds)

- *The Alliance for Benzodiazepine Best Practices*

- The podcast *Benzodiazepine Awareness* with Geraldine Burns

- The podcast *The Benzo Free Podcast* with D E Foster

- The podcast *The Anxious Truth* by Drew Linsalata

- The *Ashton Manual* – available for free on the Benzodiazepine Information Coalition website (a guide for safe tapering)

- *www.benzobookreview.com* – A website where you can obtain a soft bound copy of the *Ashton Manual* as well as various other books pertaining to benzodiazepines

- The Council for Evidence-Based Psychiatry – www.cepuk.org

- Dr. Jennifer Leigh – author of blog *Benzo Withdrawal Help* and Benzo Coach

- Chris Paige, LCSW – Coach/therapist and benzodiazepine injury survivor

- David Powers – Coach and author of *The Powers Manual*; YouTube videos

- Michael Priebe – *The Lovely Grind* blog/website/coaching; YouTube videos

- The podcast *Recovery: The Heroes Journey* by Dr. Patricia Halligan

- Paige Pradko, LPC – Website and YouTube videos; online programs for Health Anxiety and OCD symptoms

- Psychology Today blog: *Living with a Sticky Mind* by Dr. Seif & Dr. Winston

- The Daily Stoic – a daily free email you can sign up for by Ryan Holiday

- Shaun O'Connor: www.dpmanual.com

- Michelle Cavanaugh and Aida Beco – DARE coaches (YouTube videos)

- Shaun O'Connor: www.thedpmanual.com

- Jordan Hardgrave – Anxiety Coach; YouTube videos

- Nathan Peterson – Coach/Therapist; great YouTube videos

- Elise Lacobelli – Offering a spiritual/Christian based support/coaching for med injury and other struggles (benzo injury survivor)

- Baylissa Frederick's website: Baylissa.com (Bloom into Wellness)

- Dr. Hugh Wegwerth – works with people who have been "floxed" – www.drhughwegwerth.com

- Recorded TV interviews with Dr. Claire Weekes – available on iTunes

- *Benzo Buddies* (a free online support community)

- Facebook groups for recovery from Fluoroquinolone and Benzodiazepine injuries (such as Beating Benzos, Benzo Warrior Community, Texas Benzo Support Group, Benzo Recovery & Existence, Benzo Friends, Fluoroquinolone Toxicity 24/7 Live Chat Group, etc.)

- Kat Cederberg – Coach/K-Psych; experienced withdrawal off multiple psych meds; offers a free 30-min discovery call; www.thepowerofyoullc.com

- *Surviving Antidepressants*– free online support for withdrawing from antidepressants

- *Medicating Normal*: A documentary www.medicatingnormal.com/resources

- *As Prescribed:* A documentary www.asprescribedfilm.com

- Safestdrug.org

- YouTube videos by Dr. Anna Lembke

Again, this list is certainly not exhaustive, but it is a good place to begin.

Please be sure to follow me on Instagram and YouTube at Jenniferswanphd

Learn more on my website at www.jenniferswanphd.com

I wish you all the best!

Jennifer Swantkowski, PhD, LCSW

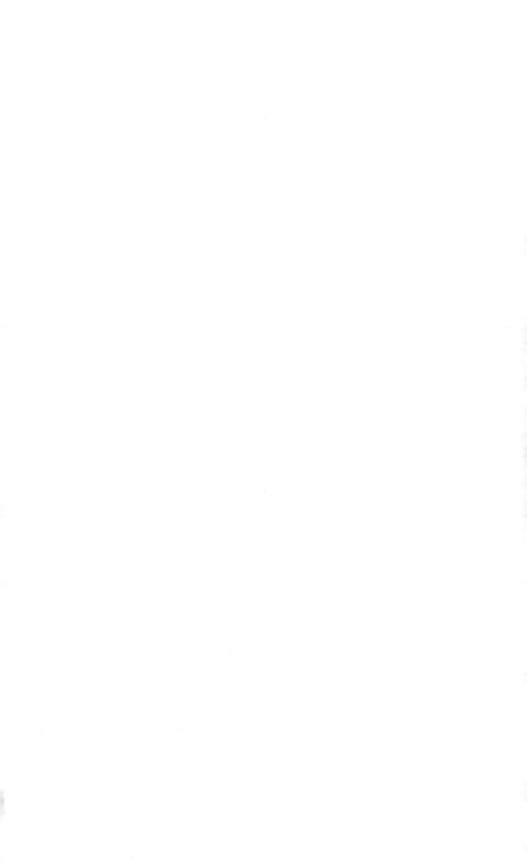

Printed in Great Britain
by Amazon

29324181R00121